W9-CIQ-243

THE
GOLFER'S
BOOK OF
Yoga

THE
GOLFER'S
BOOK OF

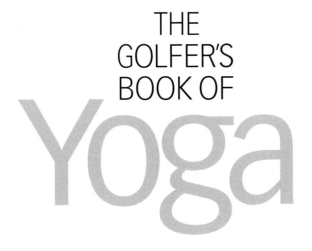

Yoga

Bring Your Game to the Next Level

by **Drew Greenland**

The *Golfer's Book of Yoga* Copyright ©2002 by Drew Greenland. All rights reserved. Printed in Spain. No part of this book may be reproduced or transmitted in any form or by any means, electronic or mechanical, including photocopying, recording or by an information storage retrieval system, without written permission from the publisher. For more information address Riverway Publishing, 145 West 67th Street, Suite 38A, New York, New York 10023.

This book may be purchased in quantity for promotional use for special sales. For information, please write to: Riverway Publishing, 145 West 67th Street, Suite 38A, New York, New York 10023 or email agreenland@aol.com.

This book is not intended as medical advice. Not all the exercises may be appropriate for all people. If you have any questions you should consult with your medical advisor or healthcare professional before starting the practices outlined in this book. The author and publisher disclaim any and all liability arising directly or indirectly from this book.

Library of Congress Control Number 2001119293

First Edition
ISBN #0-9714698-0-6

Co-published by:

The American Golfer, Inc.
200 Railroad Avenue
Greenwich, Connecticut 06830
203-862-9720 (tel)
203-862-9724 (fax)
imd@aol.com

Riverway Publishing
145 West 67th Street, Suite 38A
New York, New York 10023
212-874-5586 (tel)
agreenland@aol.com

Designed by:

Carol Petro
All Caps
273 Canal Street, Suite 404
Shelton, Connecticut 06484

The American Golfer and its logo, its name in scripted letters, are trademarks of The American Golfer, Inc.

For my parents, teachers and the others who have provided inspiration.

(Golf) is gratifying and tantalizing, precise and unpredictable.
It requires complete concentration and total relaxation.
It satisfies the soul and frustrates the intellect. It is at
the same time rewarding and maddening. It is without doubt
the greatest game mankind has ever invented.

—ARNOLD PALMER

Yoga is skill in action.

—BHAGAVAD-GITA

Contents

Introduction

WELCOME TO THE GOLFER'S BOOK OF YOGA. Yoga develops the balance, strength, flexibility and concentration that is the foundation of a good golf swing. While technological advances may help golfers hit the ball somewhat farther and straighter, statistics show the majority of golfers haven't improved markedly. Most top golf instructors recognize that good golf is all about getting the body and mind to work together. But this is easier posited than practiced. The yoga postures presented here give the golfer an avenue to develop that body/mind connection that can bring their game to the next level.

The tools are here to start a yoga practice that can fit your schedule. The length of your practice will be determined by your needs and interest. Sessions can be anywhere from ten minutes to an hour. This is meant as a practical guide, not a definitive treatise on yoga. You will learn postures, breathing techniques and the different ways to format practice routines. Each posture is described in detail and in the back of the book there are fourteen days of lessons laid out with photographs and instructions. There are also six short sessions presented, included ones focused on a pre-golf warm-up and on strengthening and stretching the back.

Indeed, beyond developing the balance, strength, flexibility and concentration that can create a new foundation for your game, yoga has been shown to be beneficial for the health of the back and spine. Golf puts so much strain on the hips and the back. Yoga postures bring vitality and energy to the spine and stretch and tone the entire body. Many golfers don't warm up properly, or at all, before they play and consequently are at risk of injury. We put great demands on the body and if we want it to respond and not break down we have to take the proper steps to keep it healthy. A consistent yoga practice can be a large step in strengthening and stretching the back, which can have a huge payoff, on and off the golf course.

And while yoga will bring benefits to the body, making one stronger and supple, it has equally powerful effects on the mind, bringing focus. Much has been written about the mental side of golf. The static nature of golf makes it particularly challenging mentally. After all, the ball is just sitting there. There is no action to merge in, no opponent to physically respond to on the fly. Golf is a deliberate game and its very nature demands a high level of mental clarity and calm.

Many pro golfers now speak of trying to stay in the present, taking it one shot at a time. Staying in the present is a good idea: but how? With a little examination it becomes clear. Obviously the body is always in the present. It is the mind that wanders, keeping us from the business at hand. So the issue is how do we keep the mind in the present moment and not dancing in a distracting manner? Awareness of the breath is the means to keep the mind in the present. By bringing our attention to the long flow of the breath the mind begins to quiet.

It is with this attention that yoga develops concentration. It is not simply stretching with exotic names and a colorful history. This process of tuning in develops coordination between the breath and movement, the mind and body. Yoga practice is a path to develop the body/mind connection that leads to greater coordination and it is the breath that forms the pathway. Golf is tough enough when the mind is focused; when it's not it is nearly impossible.

The appeal and the frustration of golf is the illusiveness of the game. As Arnold Palmer said, "A child can play it well and an adult can never master it." Of course, people have tried almost anything to improve their games. Golf is indeed unique in what it drives people to attempt. You don't see tennis players wearing copper bracelets or energizing neck medallions. Basketball players won't be seen wearing harnesses that look like failed merchandise from an S&M convention. Football players don't take the time to use GPS technology. But golfers have used all these and much more. They are examples of the entrepreneurial spirit meeting the desperate needs of a sporting community. Many of the countless objects purporting to help golfers are beneficial but the movement towards deeper change resides closer to home, in the body and mind. Ultimately, that is what golf comes down to: how do the body and mind respond on the first tee, over a tough putt or during a poor round? If we don't have our inner compass focused properly an AWACS plane won't be able to send us in the right direction.

Coincidently, or perhaps not, yoga and golf recently "broke through" into the mass American consciousness at more or less the same time. Obviously each had been popular in certain communities but they have in effect broken through perceptual ghettos. In the past many Americans viewed golf as elitist and yoga as mysterious. Now golf is seen as a game all can enjoy and yoga is viewed as a more mainstream pursuit. Golf has moved from the country clubs to urban centers and yoga has moved from ashrams to corporate boardrooms and YMCAs. They have each crisscrossed our culture, leaving it richer in the process. This democratic spirit has changed the face of golf and yoga. Today no one is too hip to play golf or too conservative to practice yoga.

Learning the postures is the core of this book. But to put them into context you will find a few short chapters before the postures are presented. Yoga will be defined, the body/mind connection discussed, the power of the breath explored and the foundation qualities of the golf swing laid out. Be generous with yourself. Let this generosity take the form of patience with the process. Time invested on this path of discovery will make your other time more valuable. Your practice will become an annuity whose dividends will only increase. Golf may indeed be "the greatest game ever created." And the practice of yoga will prepare you to play it better and enjoy it even more.

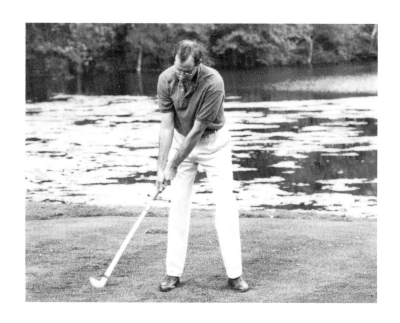

Yoga is stilling the thought waves of the mind.

—Patanjali

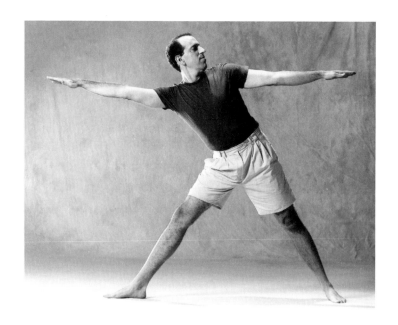

*t*HE WORD YOGA HAS BEEN TRANSLATED as "to yoke"
or "union". Yoga is a process that creates an experience
of connection. Connecting breath to movement and mind to body.
Yoga is thought of as a science of the body and the mind. It has been
practiced since ancient times. While its origins are in India, it is now
practiced throughout the world.

In action, yoga is an art of self-discovery; it is a path that peels away
inner obstacles. Yoga provides a method to become unstuck, physically and
mentally. It can help us undo patterns that we hold in our bodies, freeing
us to express our abilities. As the body opens and the breath becomes freer,
we gain a new perspective.

There are many types of yoga. For example, to name a few, there is the
yoga of knowledge, the yoga of sound and the yoga of work. In other words,
there are different paths to discover that connection. This book presents the
yoga that is best known in the west. It is based on exploring the body and
breath. It is known generically as hatha yoga. There are many styles of this

type of yoga that have gained popularity in recent years. Some are gentle and soothing while others are hot and intense. In *The Golfer's Book of Yoga* the focus is on developing balance, concentration, flexibility, and strength through the exploration of the appropriate postures, with special attention to the breath. And by so doing, create a more powerful foundation for your swing and game.

Yoga is not just an imported form of stretching, though many stretching classes borrow certain forms from yoga. People are often encouraged to stretch and this is particularly true of golfers. But the manner in which the stretching is done often creates more harm than good. Driving ranges are full of last-ditch attempts at stretching just before the big dog roars on the first tee. Perhaps a quick bobbing forward bend or a fast twist to the left, then the right, is all the preparation the intrepid golfer gives the body. No wonder so many people strain themselves while playing golf.

In yoga, unlike in herky-jerky stretching, we explore positions while focusing on the breath. By becoming conscious of our breath our mind quiets down. A quieter mind leads to a greater awareness of the precise movement and position of the body. This greater awareness and calm allows us to truly settle into our space. These benefits translate directly to the golf course.

Yoga can be a lifelong practice suitable for people of all ages.

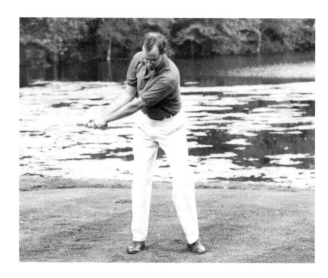

The mind messes up more shots than the body.

—Tommy Bolt

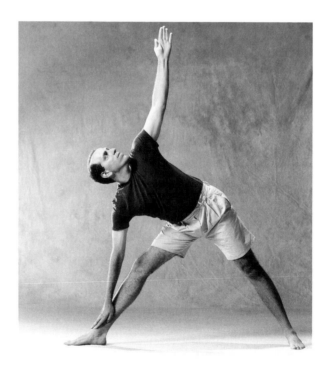

The Body/Mind: Breathing into Connection

OLF IS ONE OF THE GREATEST FEEDBACK EXPERIENCES
ever created. So much seems to be going on, so much
to think about. There is a TV commercial that captures the brainwaves
of most golfers as they prepare to swing the club. A professional golfer is
addressing the ball. As the camera circles around him, the screen is filled
with floating words indicating the many thoughts that are bombarding him.
By the time he strikes the ball seemingly one hundred thoughts have been
encountered. The point of the commercial is that this professional is so
good he can overcome the distractions and still deliver a good shot.
To most golfers this avalanche of thoughts is an enormous challenge that
too often drags us down from our peak of concentration.

Ever notice when you play your best golf your mind is quiet, almost
blank? It is alert and responsive but it is not full of chatter. It is quiet and
focused. It is generating only the information you need and can put to
use. This state of mind becomes a virtuous circle. Of course the reverse
is true. A monkey mind hopping all over the place often leads to poor shots.
Poor shots strike at our confidence. A loss of confidence creates a greater
struggle. So the question is how to access the state of mind that permits
our talents to be expressed at their highest level? In other words, how to get
in "the zone"?

The term being "in the zone" has become part of the vernacular. Simply put, I think it can be defined as a time when the mind and body are completely aligned in the execution of an act. The mind is producing only the thoughts that create the desired result and the body is totally responsive to the impulses of those directed thoughts. Of course, the alignment between body and mind becomes so total that there is no experience of them being separate. People have described the joy of performing while in the zone as being in a space of freedom and wonder. It is an experience that can be cultivated. As the mind quiets, access to the zone becomes more possible. Indeed we always have the keys to the zone; the issue is finding them.

Too often golfers feel the body/mind disconnection. As Greg Norman has said: " To control your mind and body during a round of golf with all its pressure and frustrations is probably the single biggest challenge in golf." If the heart is central to our body's simple survival, the mind is central to our functioning in the world. If the mind doesn't learn how to focus it becomes inundated by a barrage of thoughts, so dramatically captured in the commercial, that leave the golfer wondering why he hit so well on the driving range before coming out to the course. That common occurrence is, in fact, the greatest indication of how golfers' misdirected thoughts sabotage their play. If you can swing well on the range you can swing well on the course; but it is the course that tests the mind. So when golfers start wondering what went wrong with their swings between the range and the first tee, more than likely the answer is between the ears.

Each yoga posture is really an invitation to enter "the zone" to quiet down and become aware. This is where a yoga practice is more than simply exercises to keep the body in shape. When the mind stops racing the body has the opportunity to move with grace.

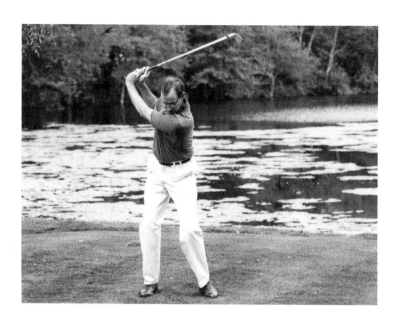

Slow down and the thing you are chasing will come around and catch you.

—Zen saying

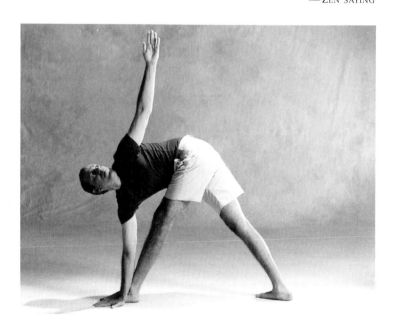

The Unfolding Breath

BEFORE SAILING INTO THE WORLD OF YOGA you need some wind in your sails. And that wind is your breath. The quality of the breath affects the body and mind in profound ways. The breath affects the heart rate, mood and the ability to function and concentrate.

The breath both mirrors and creates our state of mind. If the breath is long and slow it is almost impossible to be or stay nervous. And the reverse is also true, if your breath becomes short and shallow it is nearly impossible to be calm.

Even though golf is "just a game" to all but the pros, its many challenges and tests often create circumstances that make us tense and nervous. When you start to feel uptight or tense on the course, becoming aware of the breath can be a great tool. Taking long, flowing breaths in and out through the nose is a great way to clear the mind and stay focused on the task at hand.

During a recent golf telecast the announcers had an interesting exchange in regards to the breath and golf. The event was held after the regular Tour schedule and the four participants were miked. When Tiger Woods prepared to putt the announcers noted that his breaths were long and steady (surprised?). As he struck the ball his breath was silent. Ernie Els was next to putt and the announcers remarked that he exhaled as he hit the putt.

The two announcers were both former players. One asked the other if he held his breath when he putted. The response was, " I held my breath for four and a half hours!" Golf can do that to you, but unlike the nervous announcer, we want to breathe easily on the course and in our yoga practice.

As you learn to move the body into new forms sometimes it is easy to forget to breathe or let the breath get shallow. It has been said that yoga is really an excuse to breathe. As we move our bodies into new positions the full breath opens us and allows us to explore new terrain.

Generally in yoga we breathe through the nose. There are many breathing exercises. But rather than getting caught up in techniques now it is important to regain a sense of the natural breath. As young children we breathe easily and effortlessly but the stresses of our lives often impinge on that birthright of a flowing breath. Let's take a few minutes and do a practice with the natural breath. This is a way to start to become conscious of the way you breathe. You can do this sitting in a chair or on the floor, or lying down.

Once in a comfortable position just breathe naturally through the nose. Take a few breaths, in and out, simply observing the movement. Bring your attention to the tip of the nostrils and feel the cool air coming into the body. Take a few breaths and simply keep your attention on the sensation of the breath coming into the nostrils. You may want to close your eyes for a moment. Let the breath come in and out easily without trying to control its movement. Observe and experience. There is no need to rush; allow yourself to experience each stage of this process.

Then bring your awareness to the throat area. Notice how the air begins to warm as it passes into the throat. Take a few breaths with the focus in the throat area. Simply observe the breath. Relax the shoulders and chin.

Now shift the focus down to the area of the lungs. Notice how the breath feels as the lungs expand. Note the movement of the ribs as the breath moves in and out. Allow the awareness to remain here for a few breaths. Just notice the movement of the ribs as the lungs expand with air.

Then bring the awareness down to the abdomen. Notice the movement of the abdomen with each inhalation and exhalation. Notice if the abdomen expands on the inhalation and contracts on the exhalation. Take a few breaths noting this movement. Just let the breath move freely.

Now become aware of the whole process. Be conscious of the breath moving from the nostrils down the throat into the lungs. Feel the ribs and abdomen expand and contract. Notice how the whole body feels as you breathe. Continue to breathe with this focus for a few minutes.

During this process you may have observed many things. Did the breath feel easy or constricted? Were the ribs expanding and contracting with the flow or did they feel tight?

Was the abdomen hard and held or relaxed and responsive? Were you letting yourself experience the process or were you wondering when you could move on and do something else? Observing is an essential ingredient of yoga. Noticing how your body and mind reacts to the process is where the real discovery takes place. Breath is the key to yoga.

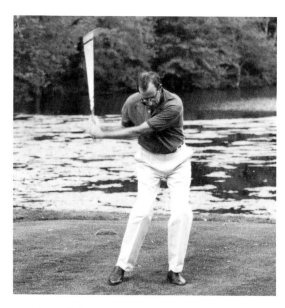

Probably the most important and useful conception for the golfer is that of swinging, ever swinging, as opposed to the idea of forceful hitting.

— BOBBY JONES

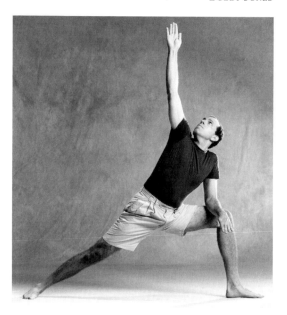

The Foundation of Balance, Strength, Flexibility and Concentration

*t*HE GOLF SWING IS A COMPLEX MOVEMENT. Not having a solid foundation makes it exponentially more difficult. With its turning, shifting of weight and storing and releasing of energy the swing requires a dance of movement. When golfers see a beautiful swing it is appreciated for its artistic qualities: its smoothness, effortlessness, precision.

The development of balance, strength, flexibility and concentration will provide the foundation a golf swing requires. Balance is the core quality for consistent effective action. Balance provides essential support. Strength gives us power. It is the engine of our efforts. It lets us project our intentions. Yet strength without flexibility is stiff and limited. Flexibility allows us to use our strength to its fullest potential. Concentration brings balance, strength and flexibility to their highest expression. These four qualities working together make the golf swing, the golf game and any other challenge easier to meet.

BALANCE: Take a look at any driving range. Many people are lunging and reaching, throwing themselves out of balance. That loss of balance is easy to see. But who couldn't benefit from better balance? Whenever weight is shifted and precision is required, balance will be demanded. Unless you are a trick shot artist it is just not possible to hit a golf ball well if you are consistently searching unsuccessfully for balance. Balance is the first requisite for a golf swing. Balance is defined in the dictionary as " an even distribution of weight, a steady position or state." Steadiness is a good word to consider because it captures the physical and mental characteristics of the notion of balance. Golf tests mental and physical balance. To find balance, to become steady, we need to become present. If our thoughts are pulling us this way and that, steadiness will be nothing but a faraway foreign land. But through a yoga practice steadiness and balance can become home turf, a place we have no trouble returning to again and again.

STRENGTH: Strength is great to have and easy to misuse. The problem with strength is it can tempt us to put square pegs in round holes, to over-power resistance where subtler actions would lead to better outcomes. Swinging hard and trying to overpower the ball is at times difficult to resist. It is one of the great lessons of golf: trying to smash the ball is rarely the most effective way to play. But strength gives us confidence and the ability to do certain things that less power would not make possible. Many golfers use weight training now and are pleased with the results. Where strength most specifically affects golf is probably getting out of the rough. But in a broader sense strength gives us a sense of our own inner resources that can inspire our play. The challenge is to use our strength intelligently; and to do that we need awareness. Your yoga practice will build strength throughout the body and develop the awareness that will enable you to better express your power.

FLEXIBILITY: No one who has played golf doubts the importance of flexibility. Developing flexibility is good for one's swing and one's health. The swing demands a level of flexibility that is often too high for people whose only preparation is to bend down to get into their car. It is axiomatic that many golfers have back problems. A regular yoga practice can help to tone the back and bring flexibility to the spine, making the back more ready to handle the strain of playing golf.

Without flexibility the golf swing can't breathe. The golf swing is well served by flexibility in the knees, hips, shoulders and back. Youth may not be blessed with experience but it sure is blessed with flexibility. As we age we lose flexibility and range of motion, but flexibility can be regained. If you make the commitment to your yoga practice, and have some patience, you will rediscover some of the flexibility long lost in stiff joints and tight muscles. As flexibility increases it makes our strength more useful. So in a way, as we get more flexible we also get stronger.

CONCENTRATION: P.G. Wodehouse, one of golf's great writers, captured well the issue of concentration and golfers when he wrote: " ...the least thing upset him on the links. He missed short putts because of the uproar of butterflies in the adjoining meadow." Golf demands concentration in many areas. There is much to pay attention to during a round of golf: the layout of a hole, club selection, the elements, the breaks of the green, et cetera. It is the mix of all these and more, and what they ask of us, that makes golf such a rewarding challenge. It is the variables that make golf ever new. But if we lack the ability to concentrate we can't meet the challenges of the game. We throw away strokes from tee to green. The practice of yoga brings us into the present moment again and again. As we do our practice with awareness, our ability to concentrate naturally increases. The awareness generated practicing yoga will manifest on the course.

These are the foundation qualities of a golf swing. Without balance, strength, flexibility and concentration maybe Mark Twain was right, golf is "a good walk spoiled." But with these qualities, golf is a good walk greatly enhanced.

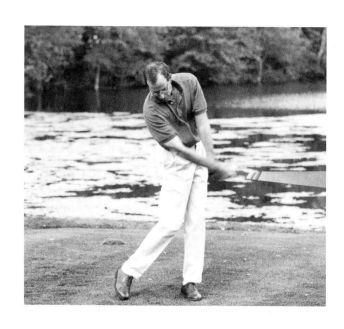

I figure practice puts your brains in your muscles.

—SAM SNEAD

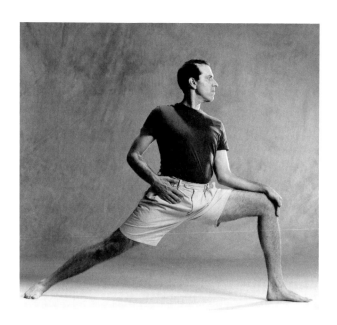

Preparing for Your Yoga Practice

TIME OF PRACTICE It comes down to what works best for you.
Yoga can be done any time of day. Upon waking in the morning the body
may feel a bit tight but the mind is alert. In the evening the body is looser
but the mind is sometimes fatigued. Generally, I think it is good to do a
morning practice because it is a great way to start the day and in the evening
it is easy to get distracted. But it is something you will feel out and choose.
It is also a good idea to do a few postures before playing to warm the body
and calm the mind.

PLACE OF PRACTICE Yoga can be practiced anyplace, but it is best
to find a comfortable place where you won't be distracted. The space you
choose should allow a full range of movement.

DURATION OF PRACTICE When you begin your practice take it slowly. There is no finish line to reach so there is no need to rush the process.
Ten to thirty minutes a day is plenty as you begin to learn the postures.
As you do more yoga you will likely want to practice for longer periods
of time. Do what feels appropriate. It is really about quality of attention than
simple duration. Ten minutes of a focused practice can have more benefits
than twenty minutes of scattered distracted practice.

SEQUENCING OF EXPLORATIONS After learning the postures, you
will begin to put them into sequences to form a practice. As you explore the

postures, try to sense the connection between them, how one naturally leads into another. Intuitively you will begin to see the natural flow. In the back of the book you will find outlined lessons that define specific sequences of postures.

CLOTHES FOR PRACTICE Clothes should permit easy movement. Sweatpants are fine, as are loose shorts. Golf clothes can work if not too tight. You should be barefoot when doing yoga, particularly standing postures. You need to have traction on the floor for support and socks are too slippery. But if you are at a golf course certain postures can easily be done in golf shoes.

YOGA MATS These are known as "sticky mats" and can be bought from many sporting goods stores or you can do an online search and find plenty of choices. For seated postures a yoga mat isn't necessary but for standing postures it is beneficial. You want to do standing postures on a surface with traction. You do not want to be slipping, or straining not to slip.

MUSIC FOR PRACTICE Some people like to hear music when they practice; others like silence. Again, it is what works for you. If you are going to listen to music, I suggest music that relaxes you and allows you to focus on your breath and practice. Experiment to see what is best. Some days, quiet will provide a richer experience; while other days, music will offer inspiration.

DISCOMFORT OR PAIN The spirit of the practice is to be gentle with your movements and not to push yourself into feeling pain. As you explore new capacities there may be moments of discomfort. When that occurs don't just push through. Slow down; become aware of the breath. As you work into areas that have not been opened many sensations will arise. Take your time and enjoy the process of opening. There are no medals for rushing. If you feel pain doing something, gently back off. At all times respect the feedback your body is giving you.

MOVING IN AND OUT OF A POSTURE The movement in and out of a posture is as important as "being in" the exploration. It is all part of the same process. By paying attention to the entire movement we extend our area of focus and attention. So be mindful entering a posture, being present in its expression, and exiting. It is all part of the same practice.

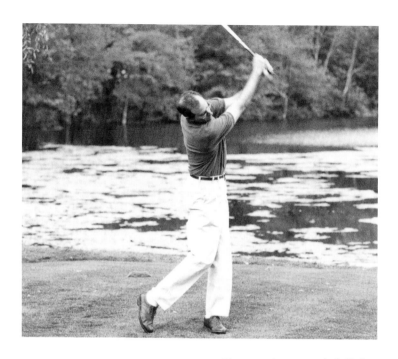

Energy is eternal delight.

—William Blake

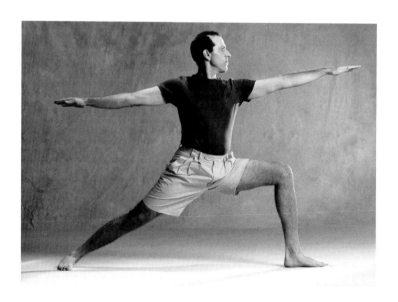

*a*SANA IS LITERALLY TRANSLATED as "seat".

It is the traditional word for yoga postures. I think it is helpful to think of asanas as explorations. Language tends to define experience and in our culture, when people hear "posture" they often think stiff and standing rigidly at attention.

Yoga postures/explorations are doorways to discovery, freshness and vitality.

They are certainly not meant to be stiff and rigid but rather supple and alive. So think of the word posture in a new broader way.

There should be a lack of strain in the way we do postures. They are not about achieving but rather about awareness and uncovering the new.

There are an enormous number of postures. Here you will find the ones that are most accessible and helpful to prepare for golf. You will learn standing, forward bending, backward bending, twisting, supine and prone postures. While the forms of the postures are varied the approach and attitude we bring to each is the same. Whether the posture seems easy or difficult we want to stay with our experience, be aware of the breath and stay present with the process. One of the benefits of yoga is the quieting of the chatter in the mind so the mind can focus. This moving into focus is something that will develop through practice. Be patient. If the mind starts wandering just bring it back to the breath and the posture.

Since yoga is a path to balance it should not be surprising that each posture takes that into account. Some postures can only be done one way in a central manner. But others can be done on the right side and the left side. After the instructions for some postures you will see the note, "now repeat on other side." This simply means repeat the exact same posture, only do it on the opposite side. It is important to always do both sides in a posture to develop inner and outer balance.

Doing postures is a way for us to give ourselves the time to connect from the inside out.

As you breathe in the postures, you want the breath to be steady. Even if you feel challenged try to meet the situation with more openness than strain. Generally when the body is moving down and folding, the movement is initiated with an exhalation. When the body is opening and straightening, the movement is initiated with an inhalation.

A breath that is conducive to inner focus is known as the ocean sounding breath. It can be a helpful aid to keeping awareness in the present during yoga practice. For a moment let's experiment with the ocean sounding breath. Open your mouth and make a "ha" sound by slightly contracting your throat during an exhalation. Children create a breath of this type when on cold mornings they breathe on the inner windows of a car to fog them up. Again slightly contract the throat and then exhale through the mouth with a "ha" sound. Now keeping the sensation of the narrowing of the throat, close the mouth and begin to breathe in and out through the nose. In this breath the nose is not sucking air into the lungs. Rather, the nose should feel like a passive pathway as the breath is being drawn in and down and then up and out from the throat area. Another useful image is that it is like breathing through a straw. Take long and slow breaths in and out. The breath makes the sound of a distant ocean.

Experiment with this breath. If it feels comfortable use it throughout the practice. If it feels uncomfortable at first, experiment with it and incorporate it into your practice as it becomes easier and more second nature. As you do your yoga the breathing should feel comfortable and steady.

The practice of postures opens up many doorways of discovery.

Enjoy the exploring and creating of that new foundation.

Mountain

The Mountain posture is akin to the setup in the golf swing. Its importance is sometimes overlooked. There is a temptation to move on and get to the "good stuff". But just as golf pros will tell you, the setup is the base for the swing; so too is Mountain the base for other postures.

If you have a poor setup it is hard to swing the golf club well. And if you can't be present and aware in Mountain, you can't expect to find it later on. Focus, extension and balance start in Mountain.

BEGIN: Before moving into the posture take a moment and notice your breath.

Allow the breath to move in deeply and out fully.

In a standing position bring your big toes to touch with your feet parallel.

Spread out all of the toes.

Lift the toes off the ground for a moment and then return them back to the floor.

Move your weight slightly forward onto the balls of the feet and lift the heels off the ground.

Spread the toes out again in this position and then return the heels to the floor.

Feel the feet grounded into the floor.

The legs are not stiff and held.

Feel a lift from the legs up into the hips.

Turn the crook of the elbows and the inside of the wrists to face forward as your arms hang down by your sides.

With this adjustment your chest will open slightly, then let your shoulder blades move down your back.

Now keeping the chest open and the shoulders released let the arms and wrists hang naturally.

Bring the chin in towards the chest as you elongate the back of your neck.

Softly focus on a point in front of you at eye level.

Breathe fully and steadily.

Scan your body from the toes to the head and note what you are experiencing.

Develop awareness.

You should feel strong and grounded but not tight and stiff.

You are starting to develop the process of sensing what the body and mind is doing.

Breathe.

Stay in the posture for at least five full breaths.

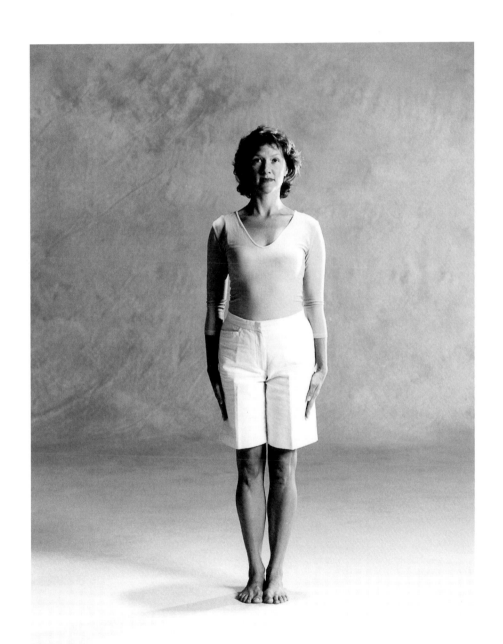

Crescent Moon

The Crescent Moon lets us experience a feeling of lengthening and lifting. As the sides of the body stretch and open, more space is created, freeing the body to move more easily through the golf swing. First we will do Crescent Moon preparation and then the full posture.

BEGIN: Start in Mountain.

Pause here for a moment, breathing in a relaxed manner.

As you breathe allow the abdomen to move out and in gently.

On an inhalation the left arm sweeps up, as the right arm stays by the side of the body, so the inner left elbow is by the ear and the fingers point straight up.

Lengthen through the left arm.

Relax the shoulders.

Now bend to the right as you extend through and out of the left side and arm.

Feel the lengthening from the left heel to the fingers of the left hand.

Keep length in the right side as well; do not collapse down into the right hip.

Look up at the hand.

Take five full breaths.

On an inhalation come back to center and bring the left arm down.

Pause in Mountain.

Repeat on the other side.

• • •

On an inhalation sweep the arms up over the head so the palms touch.

Press the palms together as each finger joins its opposite including the thumb.

The upper arms are aligned with the ears.

Feel your shoulder blades release slightly down your back.

If the shoulders feel like they are gripping see if they will let go.

Spread the toes out on the floor.

Continue to breathe easily.

Tilt the head back slightly and look up at the hands.

Bring the head back to level.

• • •

On an exhalation lift up through the entire body and extend over to the right.

An arch, a crescent, is created on the right side of the body.

Breathe easily and fully.

Let your eyes softly focus on a point at eye level.

Feel the extension from your feet through your legs up into the torso and out through the fingertips.

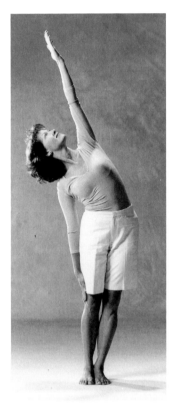
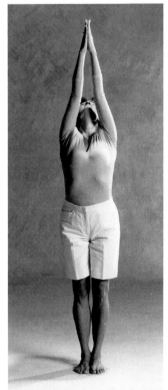
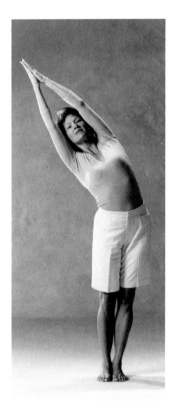

Keep the length in the arms and through the right side of the body.

Take five full breaths.

On an inhalation bring the arms back to center and sweep the arms back down to the sides of the body.

Pause here in Mountain.

Experience the opening that has occurred before moving on to the other side.

Breathe easily.

Notice where you might be tense and allow a release.

On an inhalation sweep the arms up and repeat on the left side.

Warrior One

Sam Snead has said the greatest hazard on a golf course is not a bunker, water or thick rough but "fear". Golf presents many situations where fear can poison a moment: first tee nerves, three-foot putts and long carries over water, to name a few. But these times that can produce fear also offer us our best chances for a heightened experience, for working through the fear to enjoy an opportunity of challenge. If it were all so easy we wouldn't enjoy it so much. So rather than be a worrier on the course, become a warrior and turn those shots fraught with fear into moments for having fun. The Warrior One exploration develops power and focus. We will first do a preparation posture and then come up to the full posture.

BEGIN: Start in Mountain.

Take a few breaths.

Spread the feet 3 to 4 feet apart in parallel position.

Turn the left foot in slightly and turn the right foot out 90 degrees.

Place the hands on the hips.

Rotate the hips so they face toward the right foot.

On an exhalation bend the right knee over the right ankle.

The right thigh can move down to being parallel to the floor.

Be sure the right knee only goes as far as the right ankle and doesn't jut out over the foot.

Inhaling, straighten the right leg.

Repeat this two more times, taking a few breaths in the bent knee position.

Return to the upright position.

• • •

Now on an inhalation sweep the arms up over the head so the palms are touching or the arms and hands are parallel, shoulder distance apart.

Exhaling, bend the right knee over the right ankle as in the preparation.

Be sure the knee does not extend too forward but stays over the ankle.

Keep the hips pointed out toward the right foot.

Feel the back left foot firmly planted on the floor.

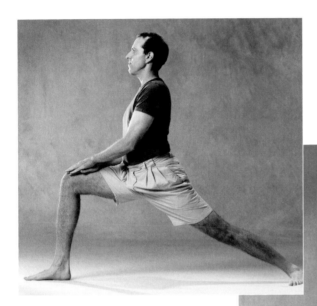

While you are grounding powerfully through the feet you also want to feel lifted and extended through the hips, ribs, spine and neck.

Look straight ahead or up toward the hands without straining the neck.

Take five full breaths.

On an inhalation straighten the right leg and release the arms down.

Turn the feet back to parallel.

Pause and breathe.

Repeat on the other side.

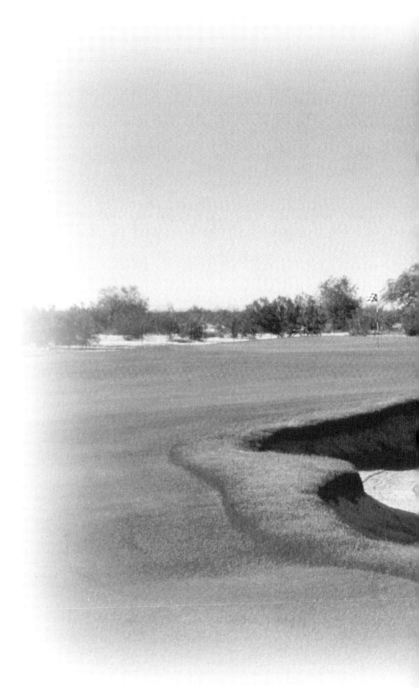

*No one has attained his
goals without action.*

—Bhagavad-Gita

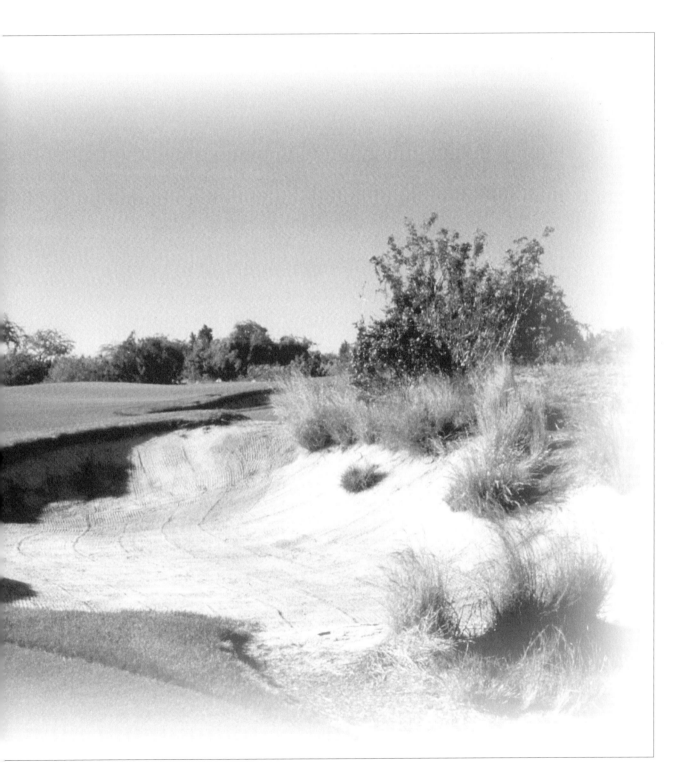

Warrior Two

To drop that sixty-degree wedge on a tight pin or nail a fairway wood over water late in a match are those moments that show us whether or not we trust the swing. If we do, the results create a sense of accomplishment and joy for having risen to the occasion. If we don't, the ball in a greenside bunker or drifting to the bottom of the lake lets us know we bailed out. And while losing strokes hurts a bit, I think it is really letting that moment pass unmet that feels worse.

The Warrior Two exploration invites us to develop strength, balance and concentration. It is a position of power and poise, one that allows us to access our inner resources of focus and steadiness. Exploring a warrior spirit is not about angrily confronting the course. It is about developing the qualities that will make the most challenging aspects of golf the most fun to meet. We will first do a short preparation and then the full posture.

BEGIN: Start in Mountain.

Step the feet 3 to 4 feet apart.

Turn the left foot in slightly and the right foot out 90 degrees.

The hips remain facing the original direction and don't turn toward the right foot.

To get a feel for this positioning place the hands on the hips.

Bend the right knee over the right ankle.

Note the direction of the hips and see if the right thigh can move toward parallel with the floor.

On an inhalation straighten the right leg.

Repeat this movement three times, pausing for a few breaths while in the knee over ankle position.

As the knee bends it is important to keep the torso and head vertical and not leaning over to the right.

Even as you bend the right knee keep aware of the left heel pressing into the floor.

Now bend the right knee over the right ankle and bring the arms shoulder height, parallel with the floor.

Look out over the extended right hand.

Feel the extension and energy through both arms.

Let the shoulders drop down the back and breathe easily.

Be sure weight is being evenly distributed between the legs, and the toes are spread.

Take five full breaths.

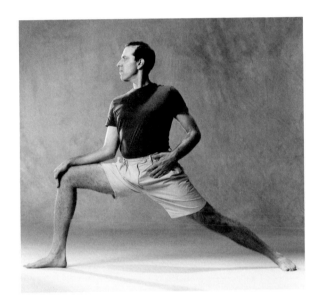

On an inhalation straighten the right leg, release the arms, come up and bring the feet to parallel.

Pause and take a few breaths.

Turn the right foot in slightly and turn the left out 90 degrees.

Repeat posture on the other side.

To create awareness in the posture scan the body to discover which areas may be releasing and which holding.

Allow the breath to move in and out easily.

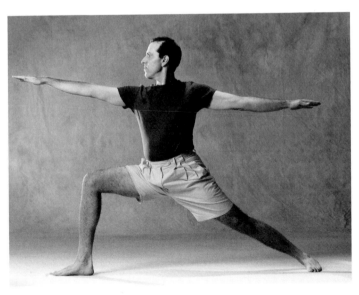

Standing Forward Bend

This exploration stretches the hamstrings, calves, and back, and facilitates the release of the shoulders. It fosters a sense of calm and relaxation, a helpful state of mind to bring to the golf course.

BEGIN: Start with the feet parallel either side-by-side or hip-width apart.

Lift the toes up and return them to the ground.

Become aware of how the feet are pressing into the floor from the heels to the toes.

Inhaling, sweep the arms up so they are parallel with the palms facing each other.

Look up at the hands.

Feel the length and extension of the spine.

On an exhalation, with a straight back, extend out and over the legs.

Fold over the legs and take hold of each elbow with the opposite hand.

Let the head and torso hang down towards the floor.

Let the weight of the body move the stretch deeper, but don't strain down, trying to create a "bigger" stretch.

Move the head forward and back in a "yes" motion and then side to side in a "no" motion.

Let the neck hang freely.

Keep the weight evenly distributed between the two feet.

To create a feeling of elongation in the hamstrings picture that the buttocks are actually pointing up to the sky.

Take five full breaths.

In this position worries seem to literally roll off the shoulders.

As you prepare to come up bend the knees slightly to alleviate pressure on the lower back.

Inhaling, roll up and release the arms.

Take a few breaths in Mountain.

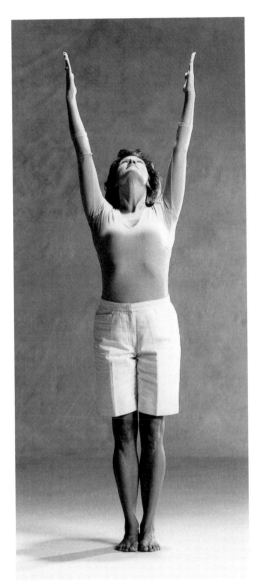 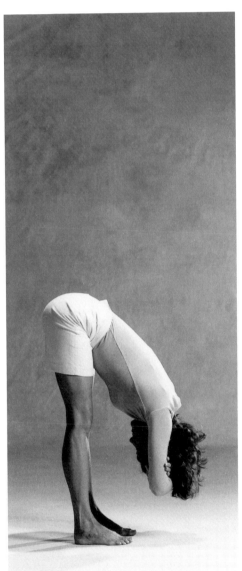

Triangle

Consistently good alignment to the ball and the target requires awareness. If you ask people to bring their feet together in a parallel position you would be surprised at the various forms you would see. We are often only slightly aware of what our body is doing in space and think we are doing one movement when we are actually doing something different. The more aware we become the easier it is to put into practice lessons we learn from golf instructors and to discover important keys on our own. Triangle is a great way to develop awareness of alignment. It also asks us to expand our sense of balance and our capacity to concentrate.

BEGIN: Start in Mountain.

Spread the feet 3 to 4 feet apart.

Turn the right foot out 90 degrees and the left foot in slightly.

The right heel should be in line with the left arch.

Spread the toes and feel the feet well grounded into the floor.

Feel lifted through the spine and note the space between the hips and ribs.

On an inhalation lift the arms with palms facing down to shoulder height and parallel to the floor.

Keeping lifted and open through the right side extend the arms out to the right so the right shoulder is moving out over the right foot.

Then allow the right arm to rotate down and the left arm rotate up like two arms of a clock.

Bring the right hand to the knee, shin or ankle.

Let the arms be fully extended and feel the energy through the arms.

Turn the head up and look to the left hand.

Rotate the chest open and have the torso in line with the right leg.

If the neck feels discomfort as you look up simply look down at the right foot.

Keep the fingers of the left hand together and pointing upward.

Be sure the outside of the left foot remains grounded.

Try to keep the legs straight and focus awareness on the breath.

Take five full breaths in this position.

On an inhalation lift up, rotating the arms back to parallel with the ground.

Bring the arms down to your sides and bring the feet to parallel.

Pause and take a breath.

Turn and repeat on the other side.

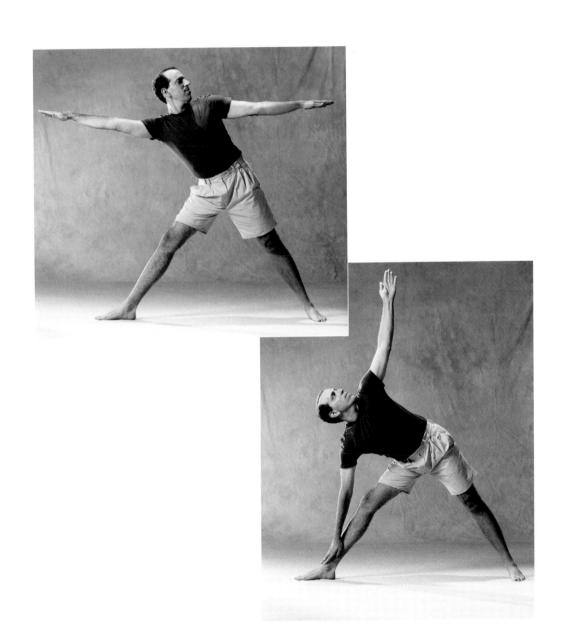

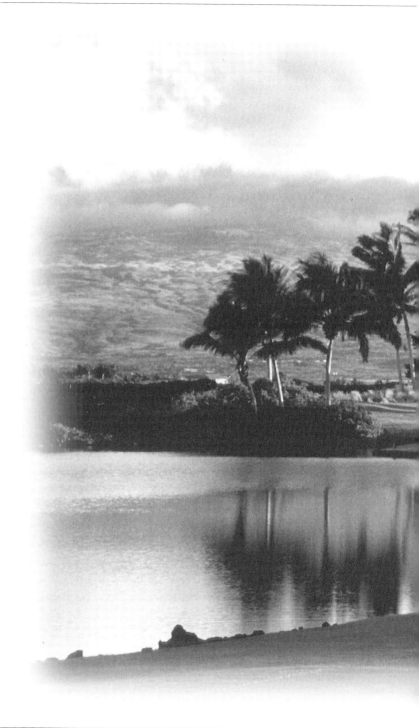

*Approach the
golf course as a friend,
not an enemy.*

— ARNOLD PALMER

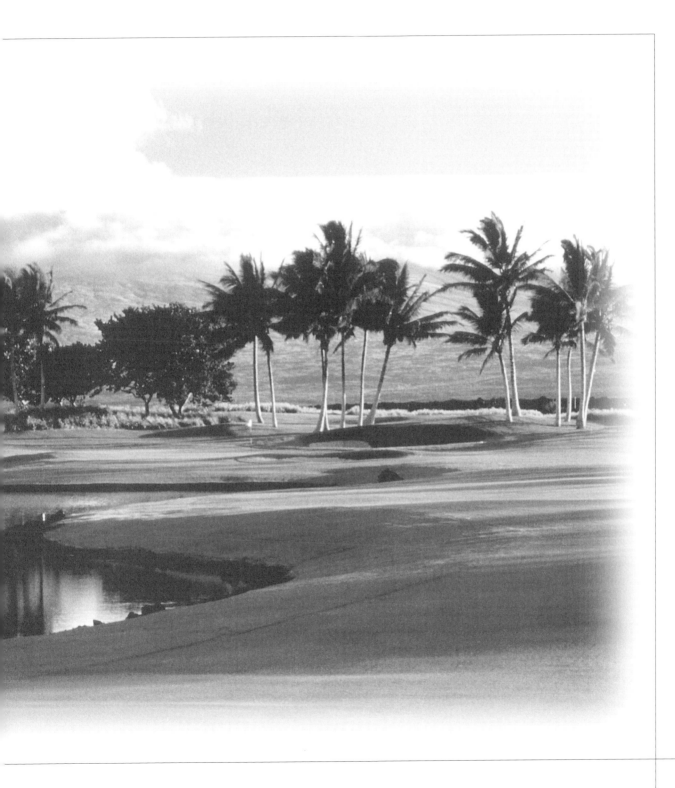

Reverse Triangle

As a young man, Ray Floyd was struggling with his swing. He had the opportunity to ask Sam Snead what he considered to be the secret of the golf swing. Snead reportedly looked around to make sure no one was listening and said, "Turn, Junior." The best directions are the simplest.

Flexibility is the key to a good turn. The more flexible you become the more comfortable you'll be making the turn. The Reverse Triangle mirrors the turn.

BEGIN: Start in Mountain.

Step the feet 3 feet apart.

Turn the right foot out 90 degrees and the left foot in slightly more than 45 degrees.

Square the hips facing forward toward the right foot.

Lift the toes up slightly and spread them out as you return them to the ground.

Ground the heels into the ground as you lift up through the legs.

Roll the shoulders down the back and open the chest.

Inhaling, raise the left arm so the fingertips point directly up, the right hand rests on the right thigh.

Exhaling, lift out through the hips and bring the torso out and over the front leg.

Place the left hand on the right shin, on the inside of your right foot or on the outside of the foot.

Square the hips by bringing the left hip forward.

Continue to breath easily.

Bring awareness to your feet; allow them to feel grounded.

Bring awareness to the area just below the navel.

With awareness in your feet and core, lift the right arm up, fingers together and the hand extended.

Revolve the hips and torso.

Allow the shoulders to drop down the back and feel the energy moving through the extended arms.

Look up at the right hand.

Stay in the position for five full breaths.

On an exhalation release the right arm down.

Inhaling, lift up to a standing position.

Turn the feet to parallel.

Pause for a moment.

Repeat on the left side.

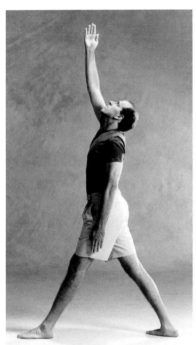

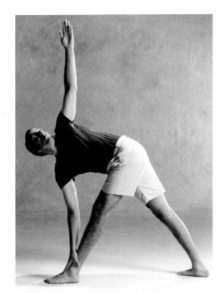

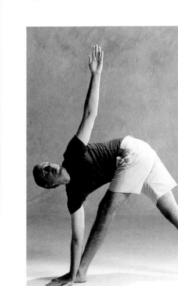

Tree

Trees are inspiring and beautiful. They simultaneously grow down into the earth via their root system and up towards the sky through their trunk and branches. That example of grounding into the earth while at the same time lifting energetically is central to many Yoga postures.

If you play on a links or desert course trees are not central to your landscape of golf. But to those who play on parkland-style courses, trees in many ways define the experience. They create borders for landing areas, become obstacles for recovery shots and add a beauty and quiet. A good practice on the course is to take a moment and enjoy the beauty. By appreciating the surroundings we become calmer and more able to enjoy our time on the course.

The Tree posture is about developing balance and concentration. By practicing Tree we learn to focus. We will first do a knee-to-chest preparation and then do the full posture. If you want to come down and pause after the preparation, do so. Whatever you are doing in your yoga practice, don't strain.

Begin: Start in Mountain.

Lift the toes up and spread them back down.

Feel grounded through the feet, like a tree rooted into the earth.

Breathe easily.

Gently shift your weight into your left foot while keeping the left hip from swaying out.

Inhaling, lift your right foot off the ground and bend the right knee into the chest.

Bring your hands to the right knee, interlock the fingers and pull the knee into the chest.

Relax the neck and shoulders.

Gaze out at a point at eye level.

Feel both grounded and lifted simultaneously.

Take five full breaths here or continue with the full posture.

● ● ●

Release the left arm, turn the right knee out and take hold of the right ankle or shin with the right hand.

Draw the right knee back.

Bring the right foot into the left inner thigh and press the foot into the thigh.

Feel firm pressure of the right foot into the thigh as the thigh presses back into the foot.

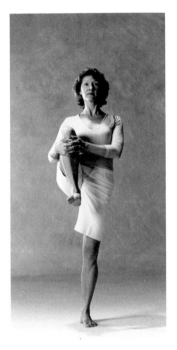

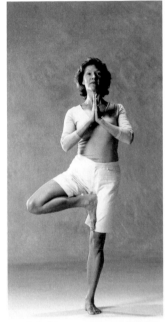

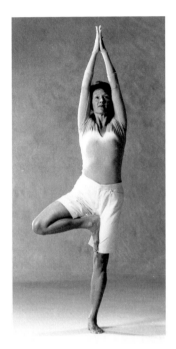

Bring the hands together at the heart area.

Breathe easily and gaze at the point at eye level.

You will be able to keep balance in the posture by breathing and maintaining focus with the eyes.

• • •

Now keeping the hands pressed together raise the arms above the head.

If it is not possible at first to bring the palms together, simply raise the arms over the head in parallel position.

Stretch the arms, hands and sides of the body up.

Continue to gaze out at a point at eye level and take five full breaths.

Bring the hands back to the heart.

Release the arms to the sides of the body and return the feet to parallel on the ground.

Pause in Mountain and take a few breaths.

Repeat on the other side.

As you learn Tree you may find it helpful to practice near a wall for support. To do this stand one arm's length from a wall. Extend the wall side arm so the tip of the index finger presses against the wall. With this slight contact you should feel the support that will allow you to get more comfortable in Tree.

Side Angle

The Side Angle posture strengthens the legs, opens the hips and chest and stretches the sides of the body. As more space is created in the sides of the body a freer turn and follow-through can occur in the golf swing. We will do the posture in three stages.

BEGIN: Start in Mountain.

Take a few breaths and become settled.

Step the feet 3 to 4 feet apart.

Point the left foot slightly in and turn the right foot out 90 degrees.

A line drawn across from your right heel should bisect the middle of the left foot.

Exhaling, bend the right knee directly over the right ankle.

The right thigh should be parallel to the floor.

Extend the torso over the right thigh.

Place the right elbow on the right thigh.

Feel the outside of the left foot pressing into the floor.

Place the left hand on the left hip and use the hand to guide and rotate the hips and chest open.

Breathe easily.

• • •

Extend the left arm up into the air so it is perpendicular with the floor.

Breathe easily.

• • •

Now bring the left arm overhead so it extends by and past the left ear.

The left palm is facing down.

Turn the head and look up at the elbow.

Keep the fingers together as one unit, each snugly pressing its neighbor, and keep the hand in line with the arm.

Feel long and extended through the body.

Take five full breaths.

On an inhalation straighten the right leg and come back up to the center position.

Pause with the feet parallel, then turn the feet and repeat posture on the other side.

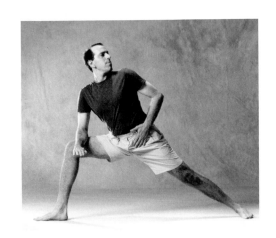

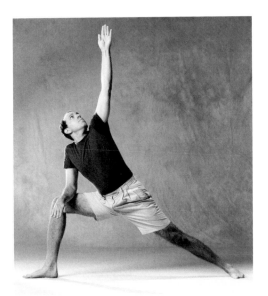

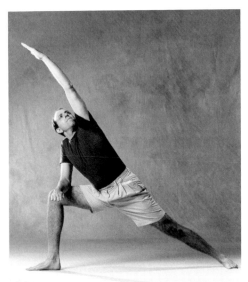

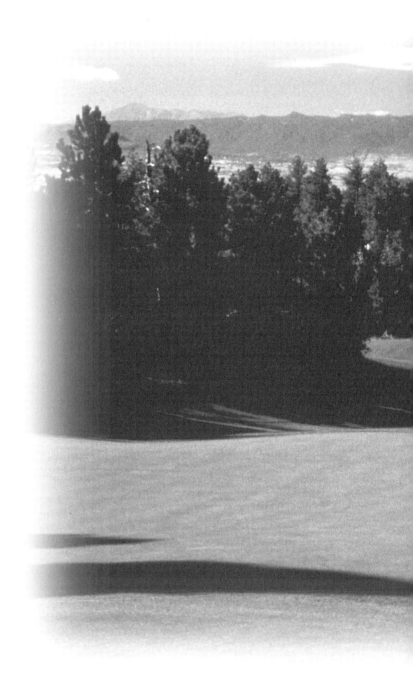

*Don't be afraid to take a
big step if one is indicated.
You can't cross a chasm
with two small jumps.*

—David L. George

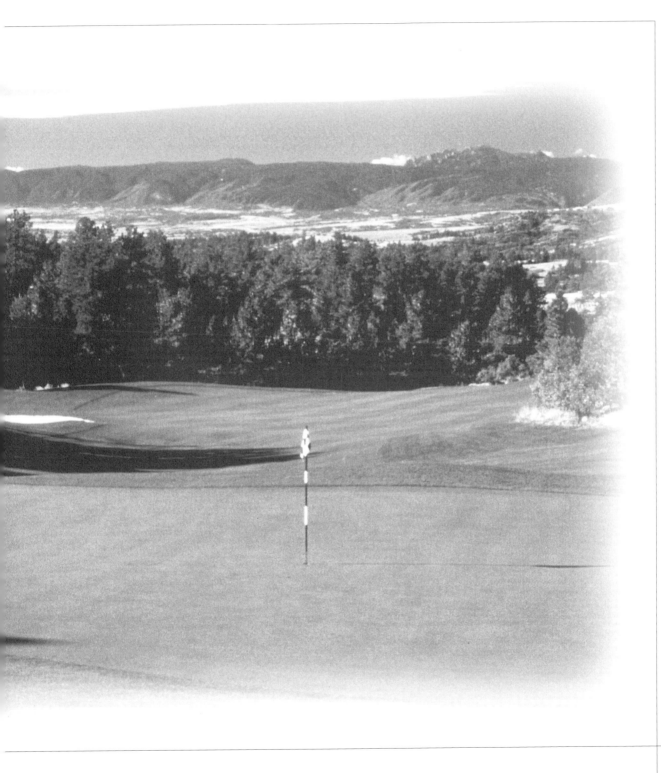

Chair

The Chair develops strength in the quadriceps, buttocks and back at the same time, creating extension through the torso and arms. The strength that will grow in the thighs and trunk will be helpful in providing power generation in the golf swing. As the eyes softly focus in the Chair posture the ability to concentrate grows. We will do this posture in two stages.

BEGIN: Start in Mountain.

Step the feet hip-width apart and parallel.

On an inhalation sweep the arms out from the sides of the body, then up overhead so the palms are parallel and shoulder-width apart.

Bend the knees down toward the feet so they extend out just past the toes and let the buttocks sink slowly as if you were about to sit on a chair.

Spread the toes out on the floor so the feet don't claw the floor.

Breathe.

Feel the extension up through the waist, ribs, back and arms.

Feel the hips lower as the ribs rise so space is created.

Feel the sense of grounding into the floor equal to the sense of extension through the arms.

Move the buttocks back down towards the heels to counter the tendency to lean too far forward.

Look straight ahead, gently focusing your eyes.

Take five full breaths.

Straighten the legs and release the arms back down to the sides of the body.

Pause and take a few breaths in Mountain.

Repeat posture but go deeper into the posture by bringing the palms of the hands together.

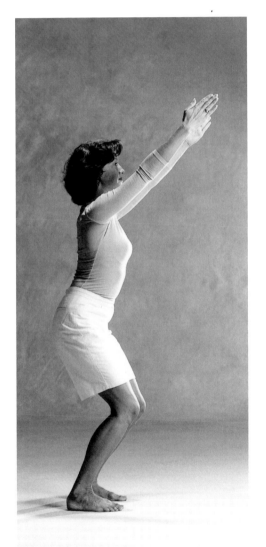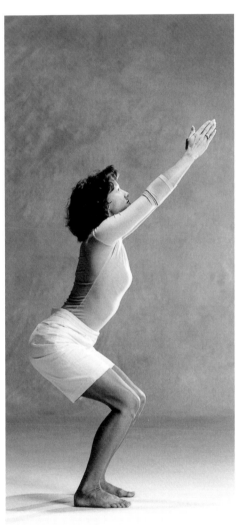

Table/Plank

These two postures are often used as transition postures in a series or flow of postures. They are simple. Their teaching is in their simplicity. Keep the same attention to the breath in these simple postures as in the more challenging ones. This attitude is transferable to the golf course where each shot requires attention, no matter how easy. These practices remind us to stay in the moment.

TABLE

BEGIN: Come to a hands and knees position.

The knees are directly below the hips and the legs are parallel.

The feet are hip-width apart and the toes are tucked under.

The hands are just slightly in front of the shoulders.

The palms press into the floor and the middle fingers and the crooks of the elbows point forward.

The shoulders move down the back.

Lengthen the back of the neck by bringing the chin slightly into the chest.

Take five full breaths.

Table can be used as a transition from seated postures to standing postures and vice versa. It is also the preparation position for Cat posture.

PLANK

BEGIN: Start in Table.

Slide the hands slightly in front of the shoulders.

Press the toes and palms of the hands into the floor and lift up to a flat back with the shoulders directly above the hands.

Straighten the arms with the crooks of the elbows facing forward.

Press the heels away and stretch the backs of the legs.

Keep the neck long and in line with the spine.

Lengthen through the entire body to keep the lower back straight.

The body is in one long line from the feet to the head.

Take five full breaths.

Return to Table.

Plank is often used as a transition from Downward Dog to Upward Dog, two postures soon to be introduced, during a flow of postures.

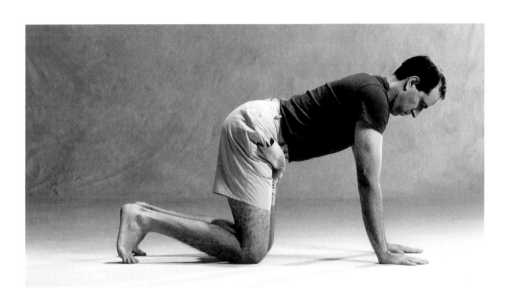

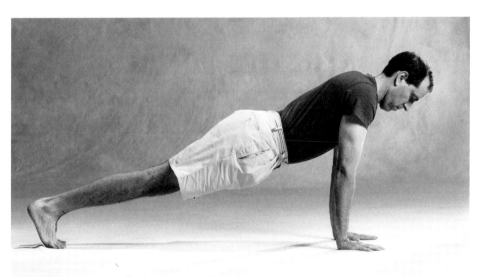

Cat

Everyone in golf is familiar with The Bear and The Shark but there has never been The Cat. But of course, now there is Tiger, a very big cat indeed. One of the attributes Tiger brings to the course is fantastic conditioning and flexibility. His coil and uncoil is something to behold. The Cat is a coordinated movement. The inhalation and exhalation initiate arching and rounding of the back. Doing this posture will increase flexibility in the spine, shoulders and neck. It is an excellent movement to begin to bring suppleness to the spine or to maintain the elasticity that is already present.

BEGIN: Start in Table.

Pause in Table and take five breaths.

Importantly in Cat the arms and legs do not move back and forth.

The movement is in the torso.

On an inhalation lift the head, drop the shoulders down the back and allow the spine to arch.

The eyes look up slightly.

Exhaling, point the feet, drop the head, round the back and allow the stomach to pull into the spine.

Here the eyes look in at the waist.

Repeat for five cycles, coordinating the inhalation with the arching and exhalation with the rounding motion.

When finished return to Table and take five breaths.

Cat also opens the chest and back for freer breathing.

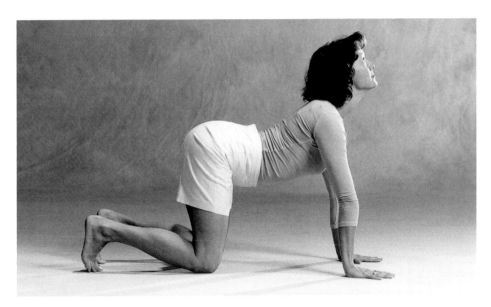

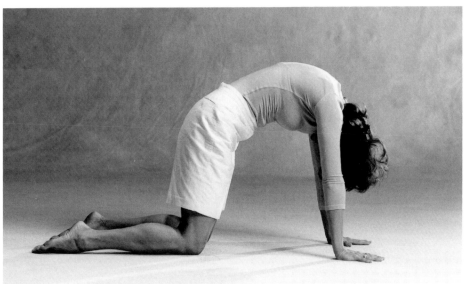

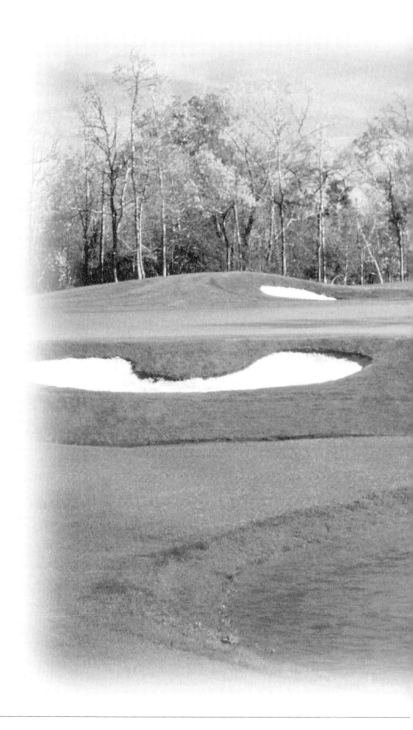

*Don't hurry. Don't worry.
You're only here on a short
visit, so don't forget to stop
and smell the flowers.*

—WALTER HAGEN

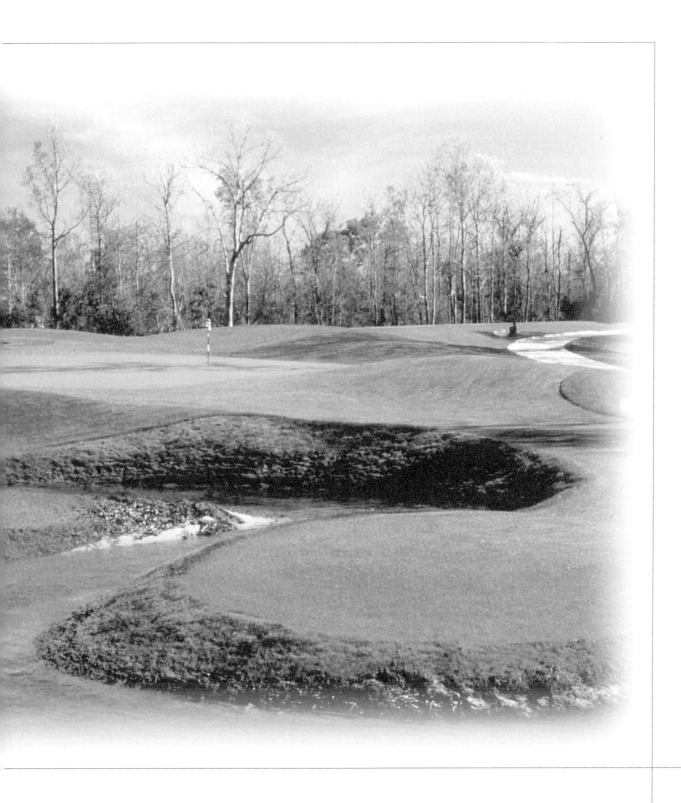

Downward Dog

This posture develops flexibility and strength. It stretches the backs of the legs, the neck, the fingers, arms and back. It makes us conscious of where and how we distribute our weight. It requires us to develop a sense of lifting through our center. It tones the legs and the arms.

BEGIN: Start in Table with the knees below the hips and the hands slightly in front of the shoulders.

Be sure the toes are tucked under.

Press the palms into the floor with the middle fingers pointing straight ahead and parallel to each other.

Press the thumbs into the floor as they point slightly toward each other.

Breathe into the belly to bring awareness to the pelvic area. It is this area that will draw up creating a sense of lift and lightness to the posture.

Pressing into the toes, begin to lift the knees off the ground.

As the knees lift draw the seat back to the heels.

Straighten the arms and legs as the hips rise and the head moves down.

Draw the pelvic area up, creating a sense of lift.

Press the palms into the floor and feel the weight being lifted.

Try to shift weight back into the legs from the arms.

Press the heels down, feeling both feet firmly grounded.

Keep the feet parallel and hip-width apart.

Spread the toes.

Spread the fingers

Allow the head to drop and the neck to be long as the eyes look back toward the knees.

Breathe easily.

Once in the posture take five full breaths.

To come out of Downward Dog return to Table. As you develop your practice you will begin to discover how postures can flow into each other. Definitely explore such connections. Downward Dog also can flow into Upward Dog, Child, Plank and a number of standing postures.

There is a tendency in Downward Dog to put too much weight into the arms. Downward Dog may at first seem an extra challenge to arm strength but as the backs of the legs become more flexible and weight becomes easier to distribute to them, the Downward Dog pose will become more restful and balanced. What will take weight out of the arms is lifting up through the hips and then down into the legs.

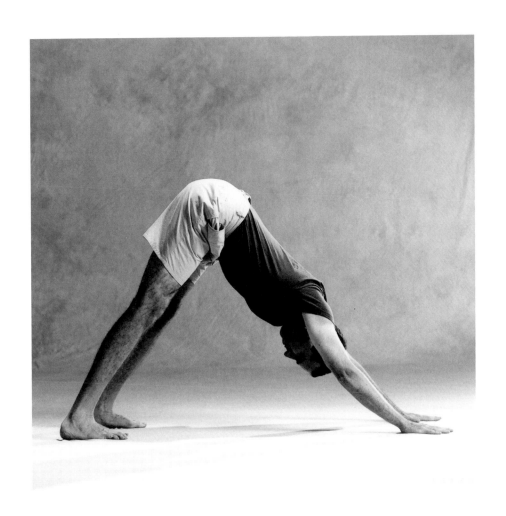

Upward Dog

The Upward Dog posture creates the experience of elongation
and lift. It opens the chest and stretches the front of the body.
It asks us to be aware of sensations from the toes to the top
of the head. It strengthens the arms and wrists.

BEGIN: Stretch out on the floor face down.

The feet are slightly less than hip-width apart.

The toes are pointed back with the tops of
the feet pressed against the floor.

Bend the elbows and place the palms down
on the floor beside the chest.

Spread the fingers apart with the middle
fingers pointing forward.

Relax the stomach and feel the pubic bone
press into the floor.

Breathe easily.

On an inhalation press the tops of the feet
and the palms into the floor.

Straighten the arms and lift the legs and hips
a few inches off the floor as you arch the back.

Keep the crook of the elbows facing forward.

The leg and buttock muscles are activated.

Lengthen the pubic bone down as the sternum
lengthens up.

Breathe easily.

Allow the shoulders to move down the back
as the chest opens.

Let the insides of the shoulder blades draw
into each other.

Lengthen energetically from the hips through
the feet so the lower back does not collapse.

Take the head back and gaze upward while
keeping length in the back of the neck.

Relax the jaw. Relax the eyes.

Feel extension from the head down through
the feet.

Take five full breaths here.

Exhaling, bend the elbows and come down.

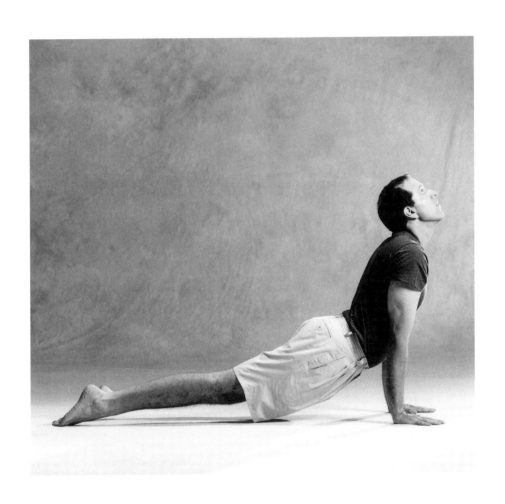

Staff

This posture is effective in making us conscious of alignment and energy. In golf the spine angle is an important element of the setup. The Staff posture brings awareness to the spine angle and also makes us aware of how energy exists in a posture that from at a quick glance may appear static but is in reality dynamic.

BEGIN: Sit on the floor and straighten the legs out in front of you with the feet parallel.

Sit up straight.

The legs and torso form a 90 degree angle.

Place the palms on the floor by the hips, fingers forward.

Bring the thighs, knees and ankles together.

Press the legs into the floor.

Subtly extend through the heels.

Spread the toes.

Feel the energy moving through the legs.

As the palms press into the floor drop the shoulders down the back and open the chest.

Rotate the arms so the crooks of the elbows are facing forward.

Lift the ribs while keeping the belly relaxed.

Bring the chin slightly down and in toward the chest to lengthen the back of the neck.

Take five full breaths here.

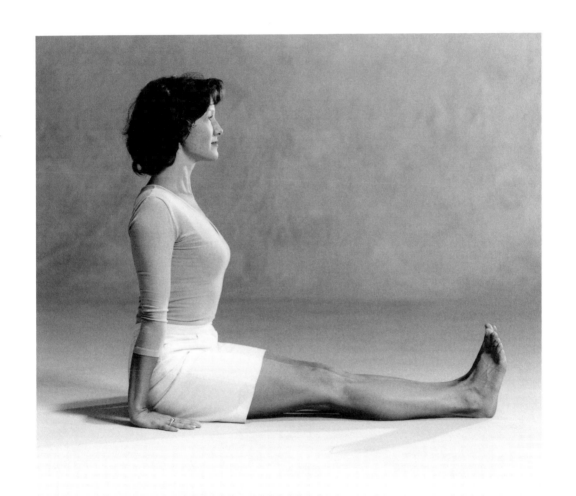

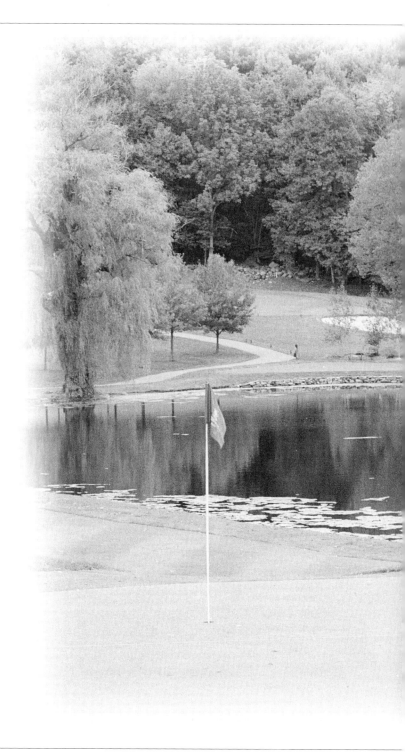

*You can talk about
strategy all you want,
but what really matters
is resiliency.*

—HALE IRWIN

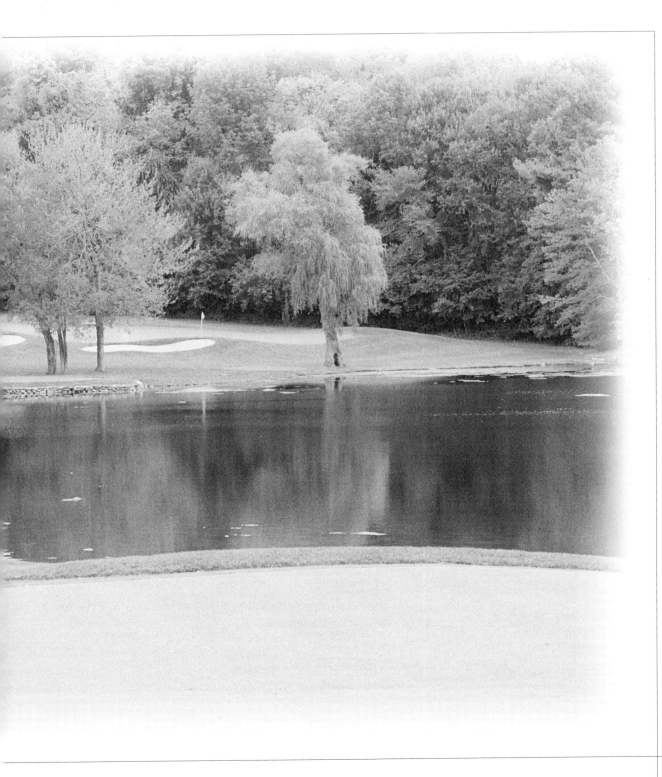

Easy Posture/Easy Forward Bend/Easy Twist

It's easy. No strain. The Easy posture is the yoga equivalent of a tap in. The Easy posture allows us to sit comfortably but with awareness. The ease we find in this posture is an attitude we can bring to the other postures we may find more difficult. The Easy posture is the perfect way to sit quietly for breathing exercises, meditation or simply a moment of quiet. The Easy Forward Bend stretches the back, opens the hips and gives the shoulders the chance to release. The Easy Twist tones the back and creates flexibility in the spine.

EASY POSTURE

BEGIN: Start in Staff pose.

Bend the right knee and slide the right heel under the left thigh up toward the buttocks.

Bend the left knee and bring the left foot under the right knee.

This is an easy cross-legged posture.

Feel the sitting bones press down as you feel lifted up through the torso.

Relax the shoulders down the back and open the chest.

Lengthen the back of the neck and bring the chin slightly down and in towards the chest.

Place the hands on the knees.

By lengthening in the torso feel the space between the hips and the ribs, and the ribs and the neck.

Stay here for at least five full breaths.

EASY TWIST

BEGIN: Start in Easy posture.

Lift up through the spine and place the left hand on the right knee.

Exhaling, place the right hand on the floor about one foot from the buttocks.

If your right shoulder is hunched into the neck the right hand is too close to the body and if the right shoulder is slumping down it is too far away.

The shoulders should be level.

Exhaling gently, twist to the right.

Begin the twist from the lower spine; then add the middle and upper spine and finally the neck.

Don't turn just the head; the twist is designed to activate the entire spine.

Take five full breaths.

Return to Easy Posture.

Pause for a moment and then repeat on the other side.

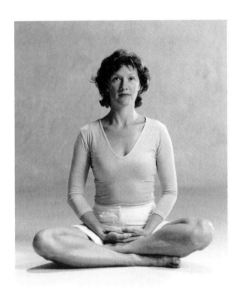

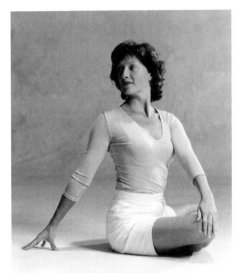

EASY FORWARD BEND

BEGIN: Start in Easy posture.

On an inhalation lift and lengthen spine.

On an exhalation extend and bend the torso over the legs, feeling as though you will lay your chest on the floor in front of you.

Fold the arms on or in front of the legs or stretch the arms out on the floor.

Release the neck and release the weight of the head down.

Keep the sitting bones on the floor.

Take five full breaths.

On exhalations see if you can release areas that are holding and ease lower towards the floor.

Inhaling, lift up to Easy posture.

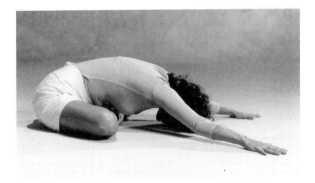

Extended Legs Forward Bend

This pose stretches the backs of the legs and has a calming effect. Tight hamstrings tend to help create or exacerbate lower back problems. For golfers this is of particular concern and consequently this posture should be practiced regularly. This posture also stimulates the spine and tones the abdominal region.

BEGIN: Start in Staff pose.

On an inhalation sweep the arms up by the sides of the ears.

Palms are facing each other, fingers together.

Drop the shoulders down the back and feel lifted through the spine.

On an exhalation lean forward, keeping a flat back.

Extend the torso out over the legs.

Bring the hands to the shins, toes or heels.

Don't strain.

Feel extended through the heels as the feet stay together.

The legs gently press into the floor as the torso extends forward.

Relax the neck and shoulders.

Allow the weight of the head to drop toward the legs.

Breathe here for five full breaths.

On an inhalation lift the torso and return to Staff pose.

This posture has a number of apparent destinations that can subtly have us straining to reach them. This is counterproductive. Bringing the hands to the toes is one such destination, as is bringing the head to the legs. The most important aspect of a posture is being conscious of where you can explore without creating strain. That awareness is worth more than having fingers reaching toes. In time as you become more flexible you will reach farther, but in the meantime just stay with the experience and enjoy the process.

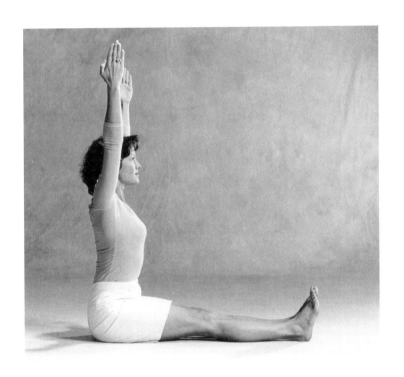

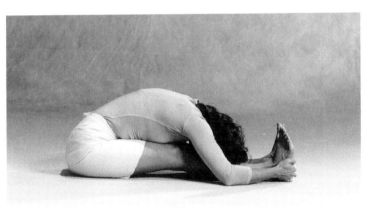

Extended Leg Twist Variation One & Two and Seated Twist

Flexibility in the spine and back aid the golf swing by allowing a greater coil and uncoil in the backswing and follow-through. Practicing these postures can bring greater flexibility to the spine while at the same time stretching and toning the muscles in the back. These postures release tension in the body and hence the mind.

BEGIN: Start in Staff posture.

Slide the right heel in toward the buttocks so the right foot is flat on the floor.

Place both hands on the right shin.

Hug the shin into the chest.

As you inhale extend up through the spine.

Feel the elongation through the hips, ribs, and up through the neck.

Notice the space between the hips and the ribs, and the ribs and the neck.

Drop the shoulders down the back and lengthen the back of the neck by bringing the chin slightly into the chest.

Maintaining the lift through the spine, wrap the left elbow around the right knee and place the right hand flat on the floor behind the right buttocks.

The right hand should be far enough away from the buttocks that the shoulders are level.

On an exhalation hug the knee into the chest and twist to the right.

The twisting motion should begin in the lower spine, then the middle and upper spine, and finally the neck.

Avoid turning only the head.

Let the breath direct the movement in the posture.

As you inhale lift up through the spine and use the exhalation as an invitation to deepen the twist.

Move carefully using the breath; do not abruptly twist the body.

Take five full breaths.

On an inhalation release slowly and return to Staff.

Pause and take a few breaths; then repeat on the left side.

EXTENDING LEG VARIATION TWO

Begin: Start as in Variation One.

Draw the right foot into the buttocks as in Variation One.

Then take the foot and cross it over the left knee and place it flat on the floor.

Proceed as in Variation One.

This placement of the foot deepens the twist.

Take five full breaths.

Slowly unwind back to Staff and repeat on the other side.

SEATED TWIST

Begin: Start in Staff posture.

Slide the feet in towards the buttocks until they are flat on the floor, with the knees pointing up.

Bring the left foot under the right knee and draw it back until the left heel is next to the right hip.

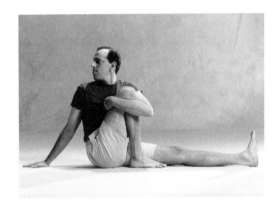

Cross the right foot over the left knee and press the foot flat into the floor.

Extend up through the spine.

Feel lifted through the hips to the ribs and up through the neck.

Place the hands on the right knee.

On an exhalation turn to the right and place your right hand flat on the floor behind you.

The hand should be far enough away so the shoulders are level.

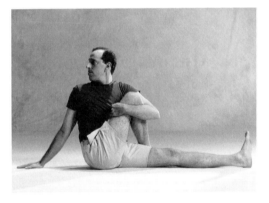

If possible, bring the left elbow to the outside of the right knee. If not, simply wrap the left arm around the knee.

The elbow presses into the knee and the hand points straight up.

Twist from the lower spine and look over the right shoulder.

Elongate through the spine on each inhalation and deepen the twist on each exhalation.

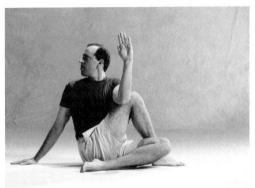

Keep the right foot flat on the floor.

Take five full breaths.

Slowly unwind to Staff posture.

Pause and take a few breaths.

Repeat the posture on the left side.

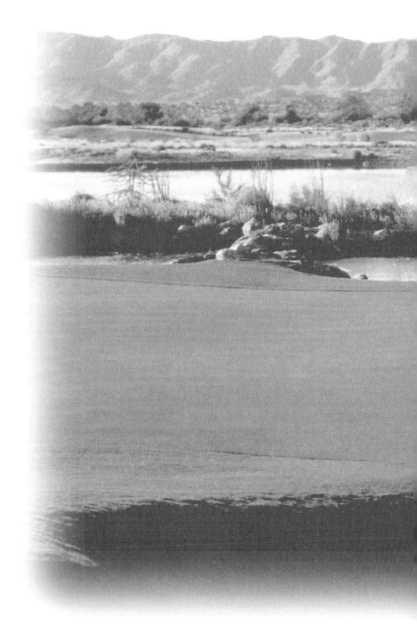

*Our patience will achieve
more than our force.*

—EDMUND BURKE

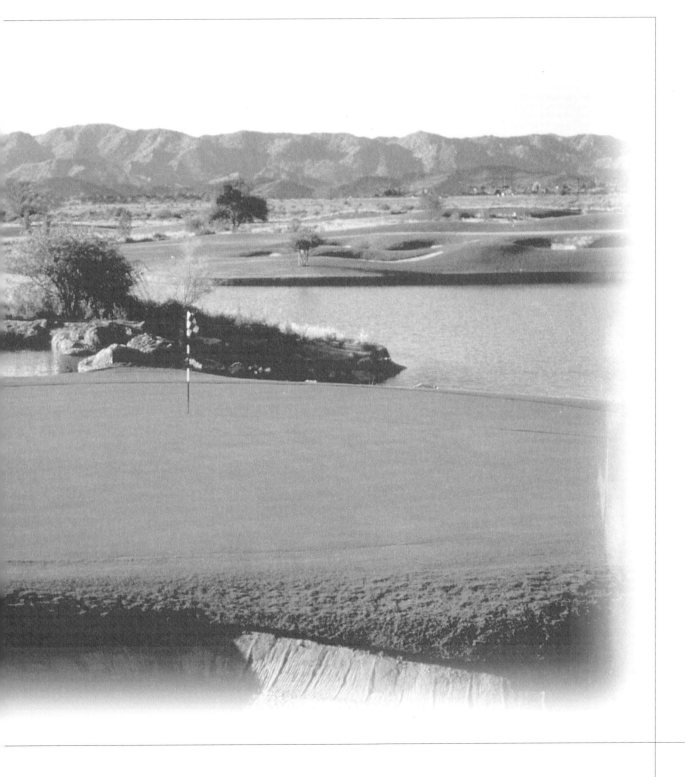

Child's Pose

This pose is calming. It is good to move into the Child pose if you have been doing a rigorous practice and just want to pause for a moment. The pose stretches the fronts of the legs and the tops of the feet. The shoulders let go and it is easy to release tension in the neck. If you have trouble sitting back on the heels you can place a pillow on your calves and sit back on that. Here are two variations of Child pose.

VARIATION ONE

BEGIN: Start in Table.

Bring the knees together and the feet together.

Point the toes so the tops of the feet rest on the floor.

Bend the knees and draw the seat back to the heels.

Bring the hands alongside the feet with the palms facing up.

Lower the head, releasing any holding in the shoulders and neck.

Take at least five full breaths.

On an inhalation lift the torso and move back into Table.

VARIATION TWO

BEGIN: Start in Table.

Bring the feet together.

The knees move slightly farther than hip-width apart.

Bend the knees and draw the buttocks back to the feet.

Extend the arms out in front on the floor.

Release the chest, neck and head down.

Relax the shoulders.

Take at least five full breaths.

Inhale and return to Table.

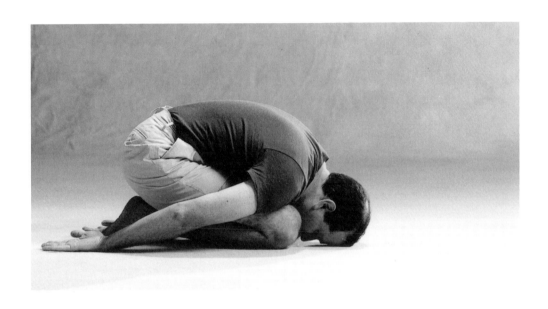

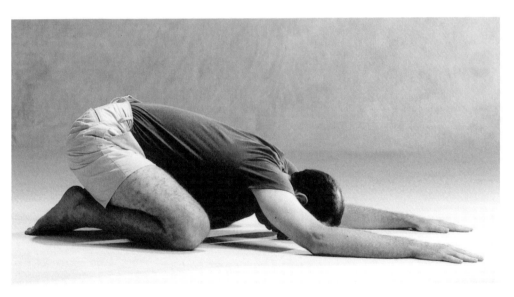

Sphinx

While the Sphinx posture may look like a last-ditch method to read a tough putt, its benefits can be felt in the back and spine. The Sphinx posture is helpful in alleviating tightness in the back and increasing flexibility and suppleness in the spine. By arching the back with so much support Sphinx is a relaxing way to give your back the attention it needs and deserves.

BEGIN: Start by lying flat on the stomach with the forehead resting on the floor.

The legs are extended and the feet slightly apart with the toes pointed.

The arms are bent and rest by the sides of the body.

The hands are flat on the floor just in front of the shoulders.

Inhale and arch the back as the elbows slide forward and set directly below the shoulders.

The upper arms are perpendicular with the floor.

The forearms now press flat on the floor.

The arms make an "L" shape.

The palms are flat on the floor with the fingers pointing forward and slightly spread.

Relax the body as you feel the support the elbows, forearms, hips and legs provide.

Allow the hips to melt into the floor and relax the pelvic area.

Look forward without pointing the chin up.

Take at least five full breaths here.

This is a posture that you can stay in for a couple of minutes if you so choose.

When you are done release the arms, come flat on the floor and turn the head to one side.

Take a few breaths here and then move on.

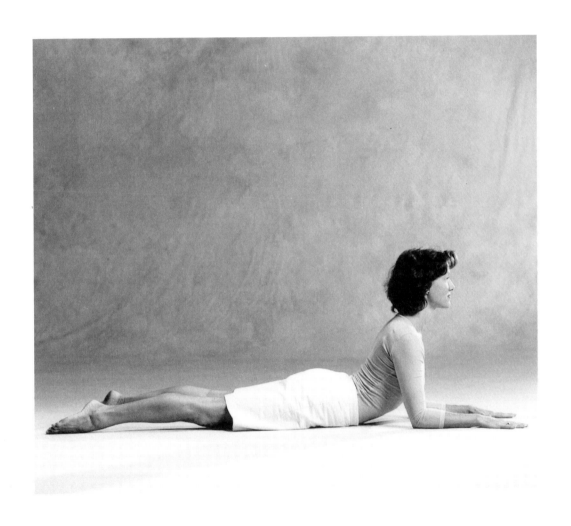

Locust—Variation One, Two & Three

A strong and flexible back is a boon to golfers. Due to time spent in cars, behind desks and lack of proper care and exercise, many people suffer from back pain and weakness. The coiling and uncoiling of the golf swing adds additional stress to the back. The Locust series strengthens the back and is helpful in developing concentration.

STAGE ONE

BEGIN: Start by lying flat on the front of the body with the legs stretched out and the arms by the sides of the body.

The legs and feet are together with the tops of the feet on the floor.

The forehead is on the floor.

Slide the arms along the floor so they stretch out in front of you with the palms down.

Inhale and lift the head off the floor.

Take a couple of full breaths.

On an inhalation lift the right arm and left leg off the ground as high as possible without straining.

The legs and arms remain straight.

Feel the extension through the arm and leg.

Take five full breaths.

On an exhalation return the arm and leg to the floor.

Repeat with the left arm and right leg.

Do three times on each side.

STAGE TWO

BEGIN: Start by stretching out as in Stage One.

The chin rests gently on the floor.

The palms are face up by the sides of the body.

Keeping the legs and feet together contract the buttocks and on an inhalation lift the feet and legs off the floor.

The toes are pointed.

Feel extended through the legs.

Take five full breaths.

Release the legs to the floor.

Turn the head to the side and take a few breaths.

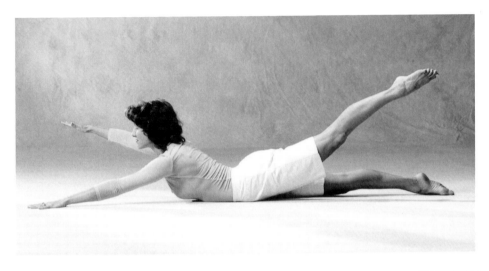

STAGE THREE

BEGIN: Start as in Stage Two.

On an inhalation lift legs, arms and head off the floor.

The arms are parallel to the floor.

The gaze is soft and steady.

Take five full breaths.

Release legs, arms and head to the floor.

Turn the head to one side and take a few breaths.

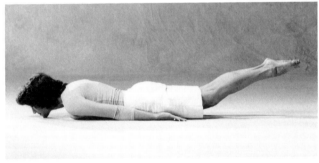

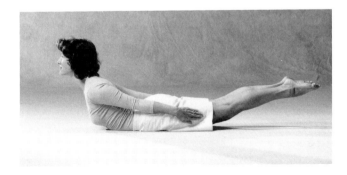

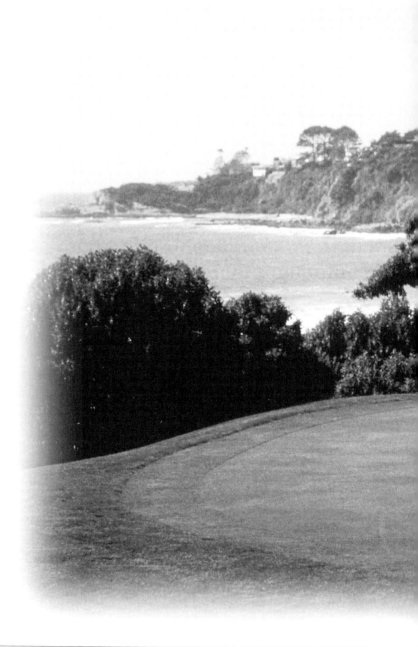

*The disciplined man
masters thoughts by
stillness and emotions
by calmness.*

—Lao-Tzu

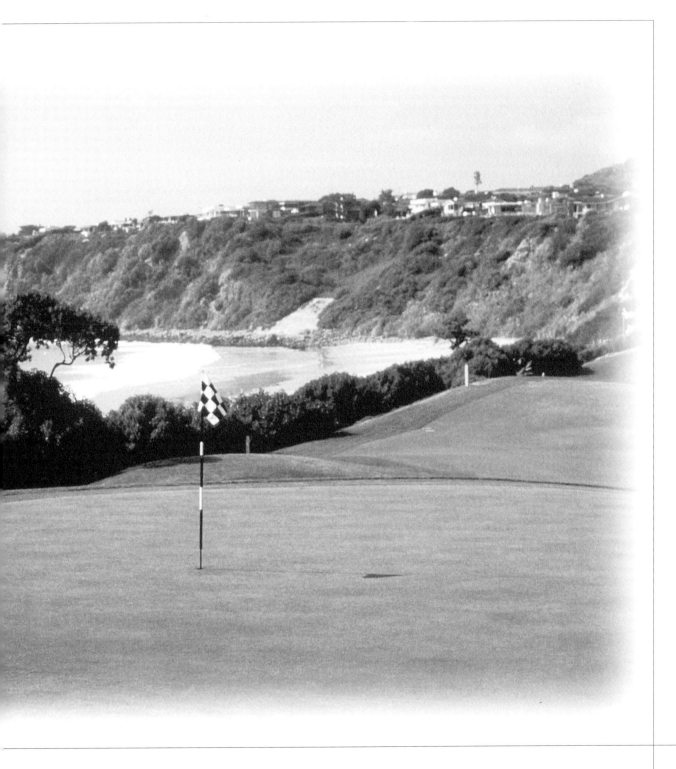

Reclined Series

Try exploring these postures early in the morning or at the end of the day. They are effective in opening the hips and the lower back. They also have a calming effect in that they give us the opportunity to release the holding in our bodies and fully accept the support of the floor.

RECLINED KNEE TO CHEST

Begin: Start by lying flat on the back.

The legs are together and the arms rest by the sides of the body.

Relax the shoulders and feel the back of the ribs release into the floor.

On an inhalation draw the right knee into the chest and take hold of the knee with both hands.

Gently press the knee toward the chest.

The shoulders and neck should stay relaxed.

Relax the chin.

Take five full breaths, allowing any tension in the hips and the lower back to release into the floor.

On an exhalation let go of the leg and rest it back on the floor.

Pause and then repeat with the left leg.

RECLINED ANKLE TO KNEE

Begin: Start by lying flat on the back with the arms by the sides of the body.

Slide the left foot in toward the buttocks so the knee points straight up.

Draw the right leg in and cross the right ankle just above the left knee, resting it on the left thigh.

Bring the left knee into the chest.

Place the left hand on the outside of the left shin or left thigh.

Bring the right hand through the opening in the legs and grasp the left shin or thigh.

Interlace the fingers and draw the knee to the chest.

Relax the shoulders and neck.

Take five breaths.

On an exhalation uncross the right ankle and extend both legs on the floor.

Pause and then repeat on the other side.

RECLINED TWIST

Begin: Start by lying flat on the back with the arms by the sides of the body.

Slide both feet in toward the buttocks so the knees point straight up.

Gently move the right hip so it is a few inches outside the line of the right shoulder.

This small adjustment will help in opening the lower back.

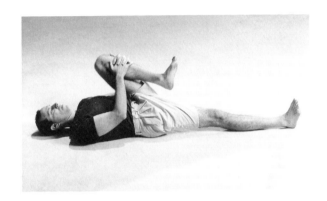

Cross the right knee over the left just as people do sitting in a chair.

Extend the right arms out on the floor at shoulder level.

Place the left hand on the outside of the right knee.

On an exhalation draw the legs over to the left towards the floor as you turn and look out over the right hand.

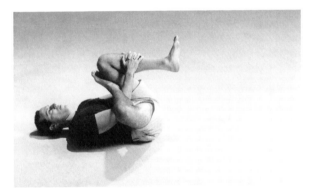

The right shoulder should stay on the ground.

Take five full breaths.

As you exhale see if you can move deeper into the posture without straining.

On an inhalation draw the legs back up, uncross them and place the feet flat on the floor.

Pause and repeat on the other side.

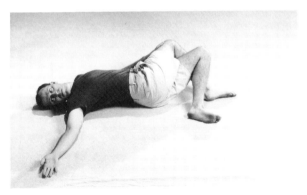

Relaxation Posture

Many say they wish they could find some. It is one of the few lacks we have in an abundant society. People will travel far and pay dearly for a cup of relaxation. Relaxation is an elixir that makes everything in life better. Not a dopey unengaged relaxation but rather a deep aware relaxation. Relaxation lets us become aware enough to truly appreciate where we are and what we do.

We live in stressful times and just as relaxation makes everything experienced richer, so conversely stress makes everything worse, depleted. Stress sucks the juice and joy out of life leaving in its wake tight jaws, locked muscles, sore backs and bad tempers.

Ironically, while golf is a recreation for all but the pros, too many people allow the vagaries of the sport to become a stress producer. It's not worth the reaction. Time on the golf course is a gift to be treasured. If anyone is play-ing golf they have plenty to be thankful for. So it is time to be truly enjoyed—play " in joy."

In yoga the attention to the breath produces a relaxing experience. Still, at the end of a practice session it is good to close with the Relaxation posture. You will notice that in the lesson sessions laid out all but the short sessions end with the Relaxation posture. Its simplicity should not be mistaken as an indication that it doesn't offer tremendous benefits.

The Relaxation posture allows us to integrate the energies that have been opened during a yoga session. After stretching, bending, arching, reaching, turning et cetera, in the Relaxation posture we surrender our body weight entirely to the support of the floor. We breathe easily and rest deeply.

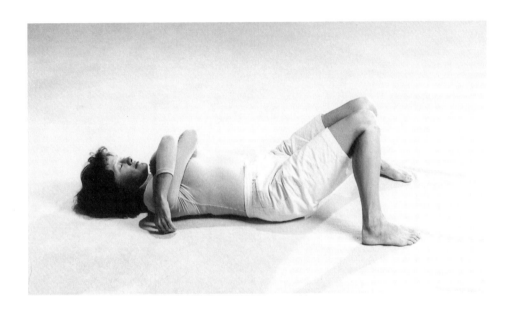

BEGIN: Start by lying on your back with the legs stretched out.

If you feel tightness in the lower back and excessive arching in that area you can bring the feet flat on the floor in towards the buttocks with the knees pointing up and touching.

The arms are by the sides of the body with the palms turned up.

(If you are in the knee-up position you can also cross the arms over the upper chest).

The head lays flat on the floor or you can put a thin blanket under it.

The chin should move slightly in toward the chest and the back of the neck is long and relaxed.

The shoulders release into the floor and move down away from the neck.

The chest opens up and the inner arms relax.

The wrists rest on the floor.

The fingers will curl naturally.

As the breath deepens the hips release.

As you inhale and exhale feel the total support of the floor.

With no work to be done let the thighs and calves release into the floor.

The feet turn out slightly.

Breathe.

Scan your body.

Scan slowly from the toes, ankles, calves, knees, hips, abdomen, ribs, chest, shoulders, neck and head.

Make any small adjustments so you feel comfortable and aligned.

Let the breath move in and out freely and easily.

As you scan slowly up through the body let each area release and rest.

The body is fully supported; all tension can be dropped.

Just rest on the movement of the breath.

Stay in Relaxation for at least a few minutes. Stay longer if you'd like.

When you are ready to come out of the posture turn onto your right hip and pause for a moment.

Don't sit up quickly after being in the Relaxation posture.

The system should have a gentle transition.

Sit up in Easy Posture for a minute before moving on.

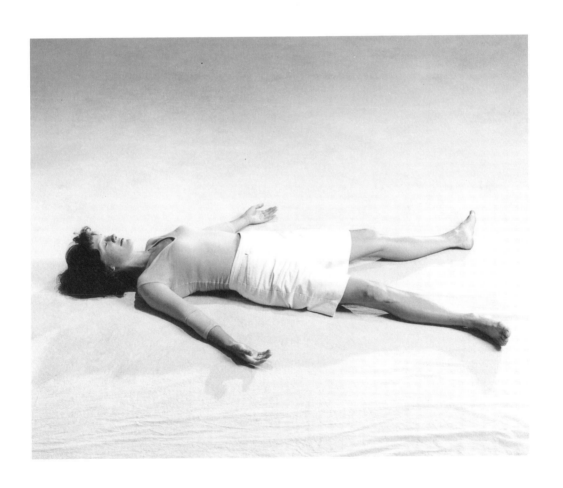

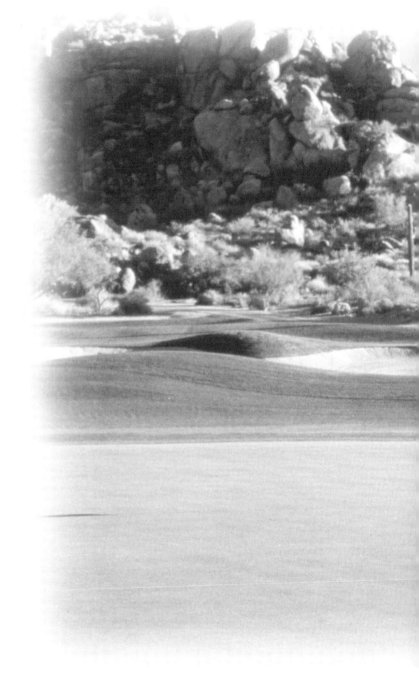

I am still learning.

—Michelangelo

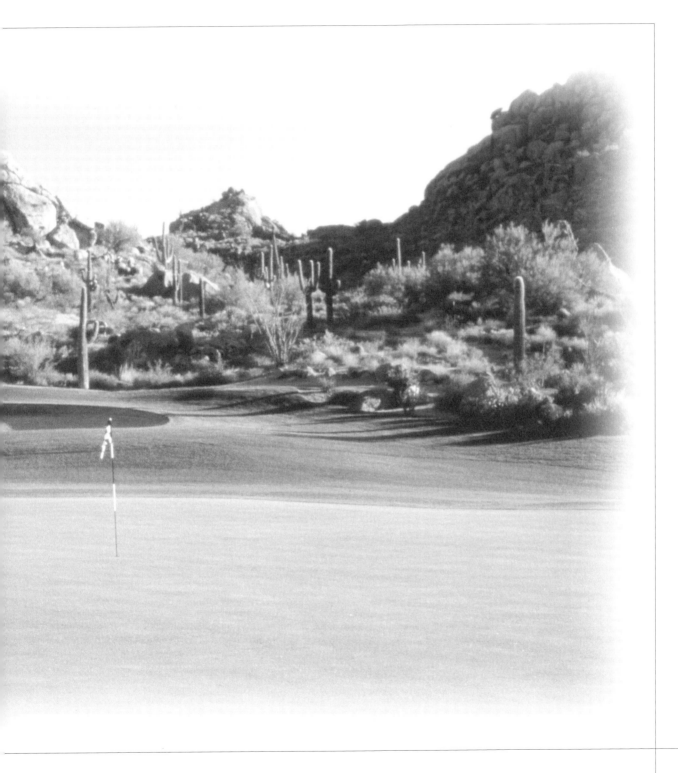

Breathing Techniques

UCH ATTENTION HAS BEEN PAID TO THE BREATH.
As has been stated, awareness of the breath is central
to yoga. And modification of the breath—taking long, slow breaths through
the nose, for example—can be helpful in relieving tension on the golf
course. Early on the "natural breath " was introduced. This breath is an
effective way to begin the process of slowing down and bringing consciousness to the breath.

Then the "ocean sounding" breath was presented. This breath is a means
to bring focus as we explore postures. The "ocean sounding" breath brings
us back from the scattered thoughts of the mind to a quieter place of stillness.

Here now are three other techniques that can be included in your
yoga practice. These three breaths are the "Core" breath, the "Three Part"
breath and the "Counting" breath. Take your time exploring these.
Experiment with one and stick with it for a while. Really allow yourself to
experience the effects that occur. These should be done without strain.

THE CORE BREATH   This is known as "diaphragmatic breathing."
I think it is helpful to think of it as the "Core" breath because it brings us
in touch with our center, our core. In yoga, as well as golf, it is helpful
to sense movement originating from our core.

BEGIN: Start by lying down on your back or sitting in a comfortable and stable position.

(It is easier at first to do this lying down.)

Relax by releasing the weight of the body into the floor.

Notice the movement of the breath as it moves into and out of the body through the nose.

Just lie here for a moment and observe.

Then place your right palm on your abdomen just above your navel.

Then place your left hand on your chest.

As you inhale, the right hand will rise with the breath but the left hand will remain still.

As you exhale, the right hand will fall with the abdomen and the left hand will remain still.

Do not try to force anything but let the breath move in and move out.

On inhalations the diaphragm moves downward, pressing the abdomen out.

On exhalations the diaphragm moves upward and the abdomen in.

Breathe here for a few minutes.

Notice the rising and falling of the abdomen as the chest is still.

Bringing awareness to the core of the body develops a sense of balance. As we bring awareness to the core, the mind moves into stillness.

Next time you feel nervous or uptight see where the breath is moving in the body. Probably it is not moving much past the upper-chest level. By bringing the breath into our core the mind settles down and it is easier to move back into a state of calm. While practicing this breathing technique is done lying down or sitting, allowing the breath to move to our core can be done anywhere at any time.

THE THREE-PART BREATH   It is too easy to become contracted. Time spent at computers, in cars or scrunched on a couch tends to compress the torso. As this happens our breath becomes shorter and the amount of lung capacity we use gets minimized. By doing the "Three–Part" breath we open or reopen the areas of our breathing capacities that have closed down.

BEGIN: Start by lying down or seated in a comfortable and stable position.

(It will be easier to get acquainted with this breath by lying down.)

Take a moment to become present and relaxed.

Just let the breath flow.

Relax the shoulders and let the weight of the body drop into the floor.

Bring awareness to the breath as it moves into and out of the body through the nose.

On an inhalation feel the breath move down into the abdominal region as in the "Core " breath.

As the abdomen expands feel the breath then filling the thoracic region as the ribs spread out.

And finally the breath moves into the top of the chest.

As you exhale, the breath empties from the top of the chest, the thoracic region, and finally the abdominal region.

Be generous with your breaths.

Breathe in fully and exhale fully.

Inhale the breath from the bottom up, into the abdominal region, then the thoracic, and finally to the top of the chest.

Then empty from the top down.

An image that is often used is that of filling up and then emptying a glass of water.

Let the breath flow in and flow out.

Breathe like this for a few minutes.

THE COUNTING BREATH   Counting our breaths is a good way to note how long and short our breaths actually are. The use of counting gives the mind something to focus on. The Counting Breath can bring balance and calm.

Two factors most determine the form of this breath, the number of breaths and the ratio of inhaling to exhaling. If this uncomfortable, don't do it.

BEGIN: Start by sitting in a comfortable and stable position.

Settle into the position and relax.

Take a few moments to notice your breath.

On an inhalation count up to three or four.

Then exhale to that same count.

Inhale to that count.

Exhale to that count.

This is a 1:1 ratio of inhaling to exhaling.

Breathe in this pattern for a few minutes.

The length of the inhalation and exhalation can be increased to whatever can be done comfortably.

Again, there should be no strain in this process.

Breathing in this manner gives a welcome sense of balance.

After you have done this practice for some time, experiment with the ratio of inhaling to exhaling. Rather than having a 1:1 ratio use a 1:2 ratio so you will inhale to three or four counts and exhale to six or eight counts. In this pattern the exhalation is twice the length of the inhalation. Lengthening the exhalation has a calming effect. Again, this should be done without strain.

After you have done any of these techniques, sit or lie down quietly for a few minutes and let the breath flow easily. These practices can be done on their own or as part of your regular yoga practice. Whether doing the postures or the breathing techniques it is always important to be patient and let the experience unfold. These breathing exercises can create a great sense of calm and well-being. As these qualities emerge through your yoga practice, they can be brought to the golf course and all other areas of your life.

HESE LESSONS ARE LAID OUT to give an organized

approach and to assist you in beginning your yoga practice.
These are not meant as straightjackets as you explore, but as you
get started I think it will be helpful to use these lessons as a guide.
After a few weeks of practicing with them you will begin to feel more
comfortable in creating some of your own practice routines. That is part
of the discovery process. Give yourself the time to bring focus to the practice.
There are no rewards for rushing but plenty of payoff for patience.

There are fourteen days outlined. These lessons are designed to
be about 25-35 minutes in duration. Following the fourteen days of lessons
there are a few "short sessions" that have been designed with a specific
focus. Experiment and explore.

DAY 1

Easy Posture (p 76)
5 full breaths

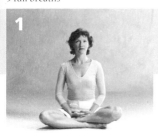

1

Easy Forward Bend (p 76)
5 full breaths

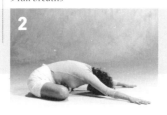

2

Easy Twist (p 76)
5 full breaths on each side

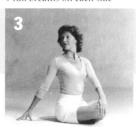

3

Cat (p 64)
5 cycles

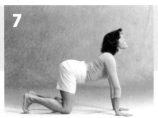

7

Downward Dog (p 68)
5 full breaths

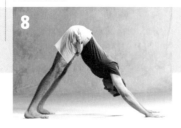

8

Plank (p 62)
3 full breaths

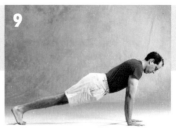

9

Crescent Moon (p 38)
5 full breaths on each side

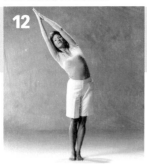

12

Warrior One (p 40)
5 full breaths on each side

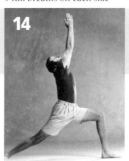

14

Mountain (p 36)
5 full breaths

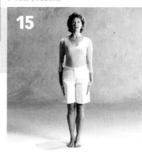

15

Staff *(p 72)*
5 full breaths

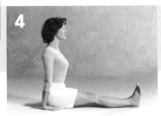

4

Extended Legs Forward Bend *(p 78)*
5 full breaths

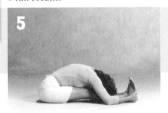

5

Table Top *(p 62)*
5 full breaths

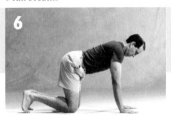

6

Upward Dog *(p 70)*
3 full breaths

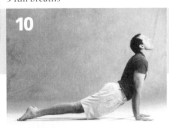

10

Child's Pose *(p 84)*
5 full breaths

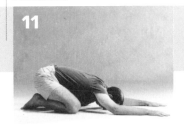

11

Mountain *(p 36)*
5 full breaths

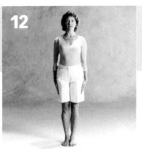

12

Standing Forward Bend *(p 46)*
5 full breaths

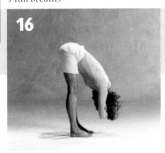

16

Relaxation Pose *(p 94)*
3 minutes plus

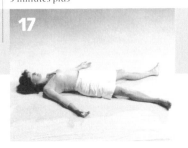

17

Easy Posture *(p 76)*
5 full breaths

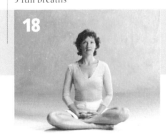

18

DAY 2

Easy Posture (p 76)
5 full breaths

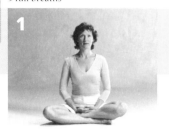

1

Reclined Knee to Chest (p 92)
5 full breaths on each side

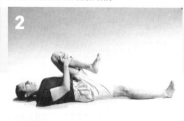

2

Reclined Ankle to Knee (p 92)
5 full breaths on each side

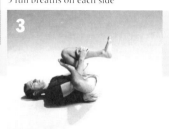

3

Extended Leg Twist (p 80)
5 full breaths on each side

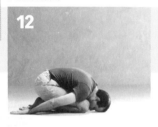

7

Table (p 62)
5 full breaths

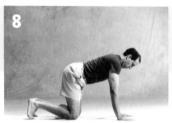

8

Cat (p 64)
5 cycles

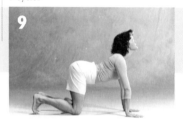

9

Child's Pose (p 84)
5 full breaths

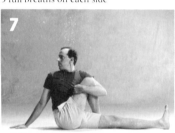

12

Mountain (p 36)
5 full breaths

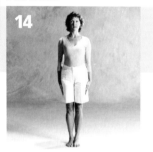

14

Crescent Moon (p 38)
5 full breaths on each side

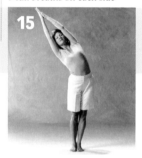

15

Standing Forward Bend (p 46)
5 full breaths

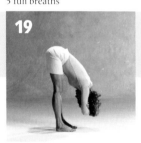

19

Relaxation Pose (p 94)
3 minutes plus

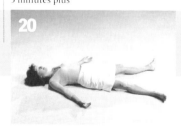

20

Easy Posture (p 74)
5 full breaths

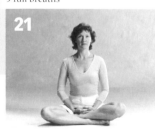

21

Reclined Twist *(p 92)*
5 full breaths on each side

4

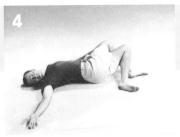

Staff *(p 72)*
5 full breaths

5

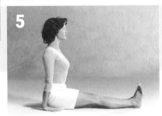

Extended Legs Forward Bend *(p 78)*
5 full breaths

6

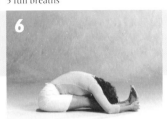

Downward Dog *(p 68)*
5 full breaths

10

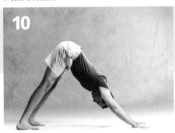

Plank *(p 62)*
3 full breaths

11

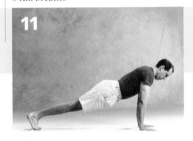

Upward Dog *(p 70)*
3 full breaths

12

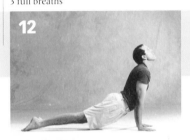

Warrior One *(p 40)*
5 full breaths on each side

16

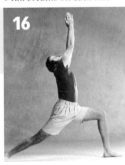

Warrior Two *(p 44)*
5 full breaths on each side

17

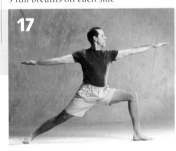

Mountain *(p 36)*
5 full breaths

18

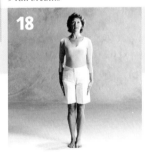

DAY 3

Easy Posture *(p 76)*
5 full breaths

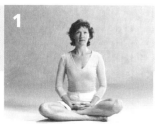
1

Easy Forward Bend *(p 76)*
5 full breaths

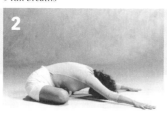
2

Easy Seated Twist *(p 76)*
5 full breaths on each side

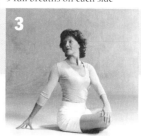
3

Extended Legs Forward Bend *(p 78)*
5 full breaths

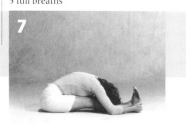
7

Cat *(p 64)*
5 cycles

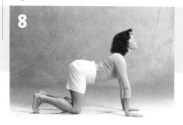
8

Mountain *(p 36)*
5 full breaths

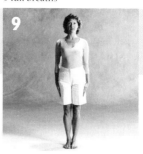
9

Chair *(p 60)*
5 full breaths

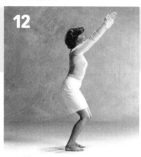
12

Tree *(p 54)*
5 full breaths

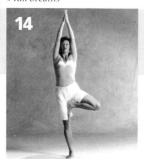
14

Triangle *(p 48)*
5 full breaths on each side

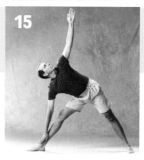
15

Sphinx *(p 86)*
9 full breaths

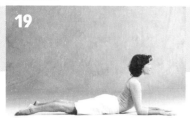
19

Relaxation Pose *(p 94)*
3 minutes plus

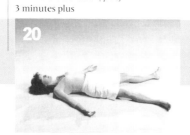
20

Easy Posture *(p 76)*
5 full breaths

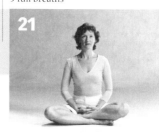
21

Staff *(p 72)*
5 full breaths

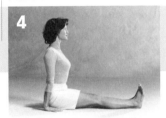

Extended Legs Forward Bend *(p 78)*
5 full breaths

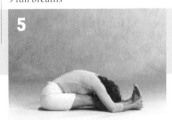

Extended Leg Twist *(p 80)*
5 full breaths on each side

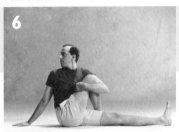

Crescent Moon *(p 38)*
5 full breaths on each side

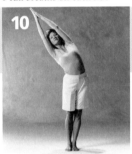

Standing Forward Bend *(p 46)*
5 full breaths

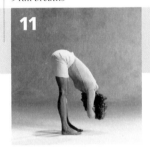

Mountain *(p 36)*
5 full breaths

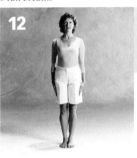

Warrior One *(p 40)*
5 full breaths on each side

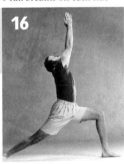

Warrior Two *(p 44)*
5 full breaths on each side

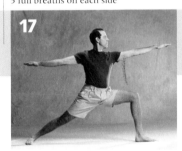

Mountain *(p 36)*
5 full breaths

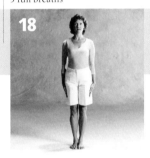

DAY 4

Easy Posture *(p 76)*
5 full breaths

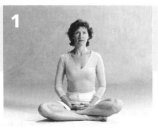

Easy Forward Bend *(p 76)*
5 full breaths

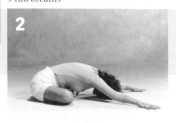

Easy Twist *(p 76)*
5 full breaths on each side

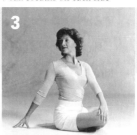

Cat *(p 64)*
5 cycles

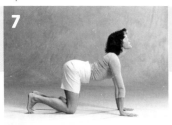

Downward Dog *(p 68)*
5 full breaths

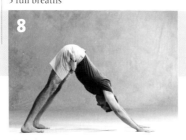

Plank *(p 62)*
3 full breaths

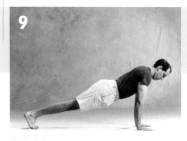

Crescent Moon *(p 38)*
5 full breaths on each side

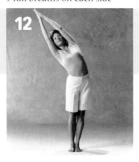

Side Angle *(p 56)*
5 full breaths on each side

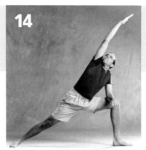

Triangle *(p 48)*
5 full breaths on each side

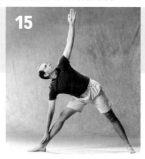

Standing Forward Bend *(p 46)*
5 full breaths

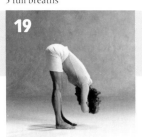

Relaxation Pose *(p 94)*
3 minutes plus

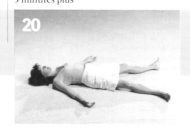

Easy Posture *(p 76)*
5 full breaths

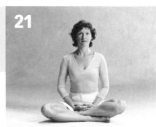

Staff *(p 72)*
5 full breaths

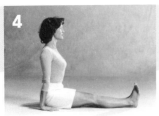

4

Extended Legs Forward Bend *(p 78)*
5 full breaths

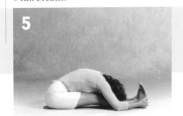

5

Table *(p 62)*
5 full breaths

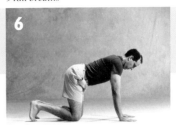

6

Upward Dog *(p 70)*
3 full breaths

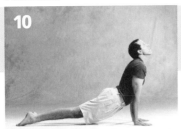

10

Child's Pose *(p 84)*
5 full breaths

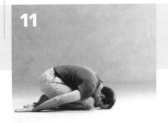

11

Mountain *(p 36)*
5 full breaths

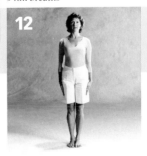

12

Reverse Triangle *(p 52)*
5 full breaths on each side

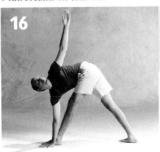

16

Mountain *(p 36)*
5 full breaths

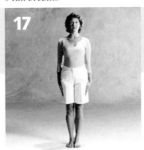

17

Tree *(p 54)*
5 full breaths on each side

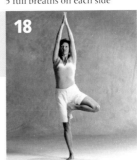

18

DAY 5

Easy Posture (p 76)
5 full breaths

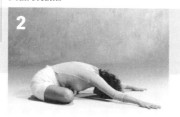
1

Easy Forward Bend (p 76)
5 full breaths

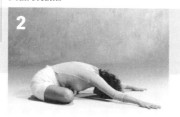
2

Easy Twist (p 76)
5 full breaths on each side

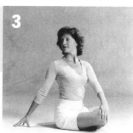
3

Standing Forward Bend (p 46)
5 full breaths

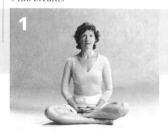
7

Tree (p 54)
5 full breaths on each side

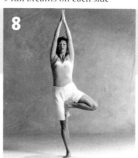
8

Chair (p 60)
5 full breaths

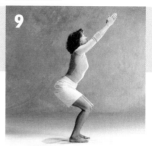
9

Reverse Triangle (p 52)
5 full breaths on each side

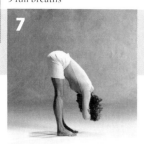
12

Mountain (p 36)
5 full breaths

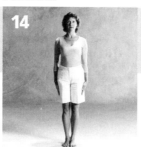
14

Standing Forward Bend (p 46)
5 full breaths

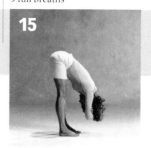
15

Plank (p 62)
3 full breaths

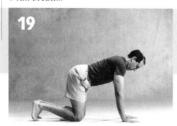
19

Upward Dog (p 70)
3 full breaths

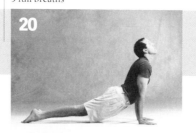
20

Sphinx (p 86)
9 full breaths

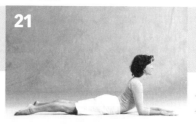
21

Extended Legs Forward Bend (p 78)
5 full breaths

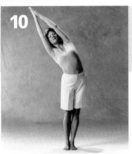

Mountain (p 36)
5 full breaths

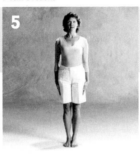

Crescent Moon (p 38)
5 breaths on each side

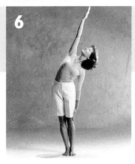

Crescent Moon (p 38)
5 full breaths on each side

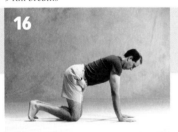

Side Angle (p 56)
5 full breaths on each side

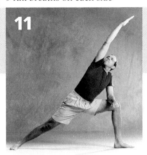

Triangle (p 48)
5 full breaths on each side

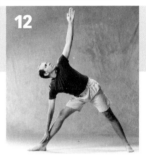

Table (p 62)
5 full breaths

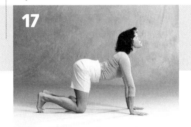

Cat (p 64)
5 cycles

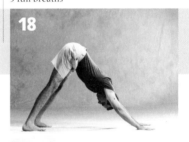

Downward Dog (p 68)
5 full breaths

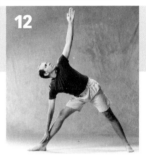

Child's Pose (p 84)
5 full breaths

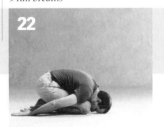

Relaxation Pose (p 94)
3 minutes plus

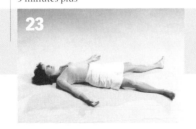

Easy Posture (p 76)
5 full breaths

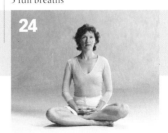

115

DAY 6

Easy Posture (p 76)
5 full breaths

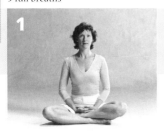
1

Reclined Knee to Chest (p 92)
5 full breaths on each side

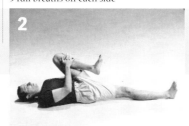
2

Reclined Ankle to Knee (p 92)
5 full breaths on each side

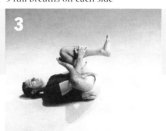
3

Downward Dog (p 68)
5 full breaths

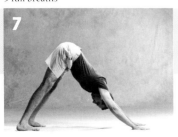
7

Plank (p 62)
3 full breaths

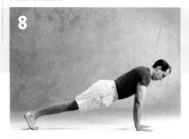
8

Upward Dog (p 70)
3 full breaths

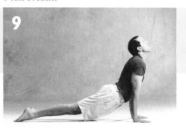
9

Table (p 62)
5 full breaths

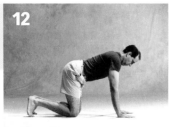
12

Downward Dog (p 68)
5 full breaths

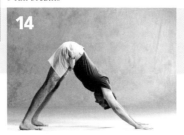
14

Mountain (p 36)
5 full breaths

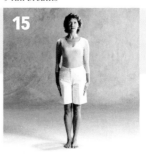
15

Warrior Two (p 44)
5 full breaths on each side

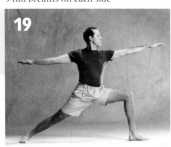
19

Triangle (p 48)
5 full breaths on each side

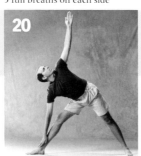
20

Reverse Triangle (p 52)
5 full breaths on each side

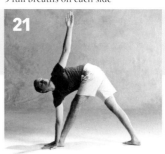
21

Reclined Twist *(p 92)*
5 full breaths on each side

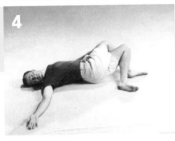

Table *(p 62)*
5 full breaths

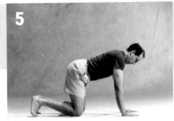

Cat *(p 64)*
5 cycles

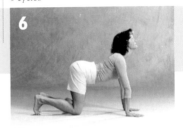

Child's Pose *(p 84)*
5 full breaths

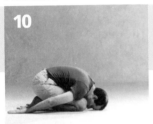

Sphinx *(p 86)*
9 full breaths

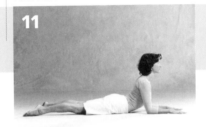

Locust *(p 88)*
5 full breaths

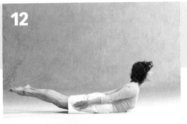

Crescent Moon *(p 38)*
5 full breaths on each side

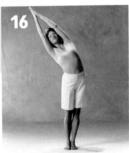

Side Angle *(p 56)*
5 full breaths on each side

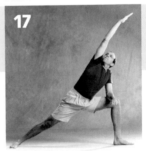

Warrior One *(p 40)*
5 full breaths on each side

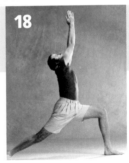

Mountain *(p 36)*
5 full breaths on each side

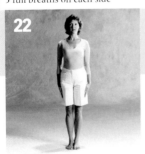

Relaxation Pose *(p 94)*
3 minutes plus

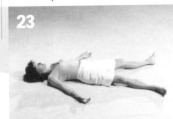

Easy Posture *(p 76)*
5 full breaths

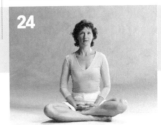

DAY 7

Easy Posture (p 76)
5 full breaths

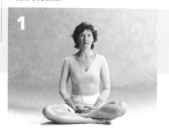

1

Easy Forward Bend (p 76)
5 full breaths

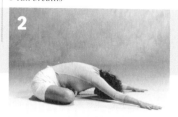

2

Easy Twist (p 76)
5 full breaths

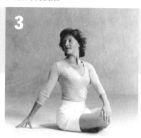

3

Extended Leg Twist (p 80)
5 full breaths on each side

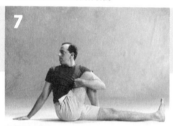

7

Table (p 62)
5 full breaths

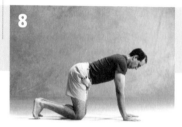

8

Cat (p 64)
5 cycles

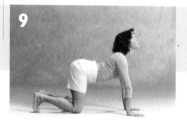

9

Mountain (p 36)
5 full breaths

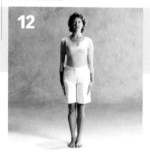

12

Crescent Moon (p 38)
5 full breaths on each side

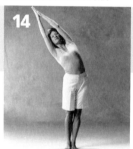

14

Tree (p 54)
5 full breaths on each side

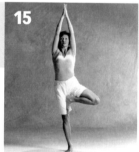

15

Reverse Triangle (p 52)
5 full breaths on each side

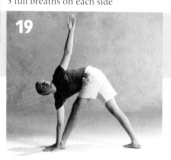

19

Mountain (p 36)
5 full breaths

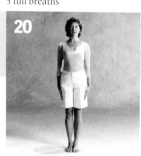

20

Sphinx (p 86)
9 full breaths

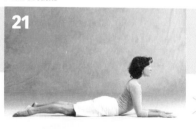

21

Staff *(p 72)*
5 full breaths

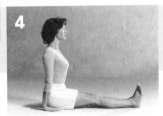

Extended Legs Forward Bend *(p 78)*
5 full breaths

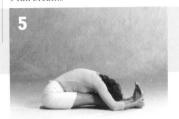

Staff *(p 72)*
5 full breaths

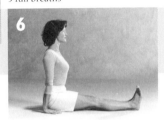

Downward Dog *(p 68)*
5 full breaths

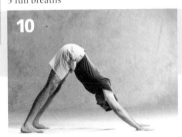

Upward Dog *(p 70)*
3 full breaths

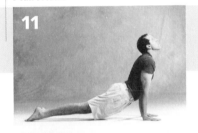

Child's Pose *(p 84)*
5 full breaths

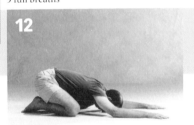

Chair *(p 60)*
5 full breaths

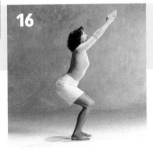

Side Angle *(p 56)*
5 full breaths on each side

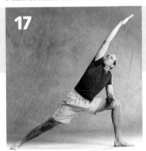

Triangle *(p 48)*
5 full breaths on each side

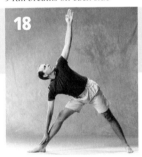

Child Pose *(p 84)*
5 full breaths

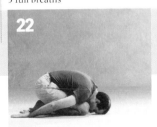

Relaxation Pose *(p 94)*
3 minutes plus

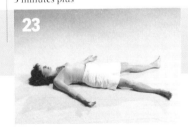

Easy Posture *(p 76)*
5 full breaths

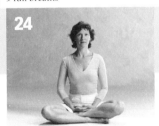

DAY 8

Easy Posture *(p 76)*
5 full breaths

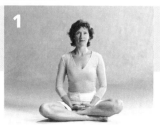

Staff *(p 72)*
5 full breaths

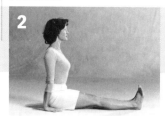

Extended Legs Forward Bend *(p 78)*
5 full breaths

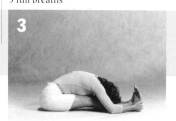

Downward Dog *(p 68)*
5 full breaths

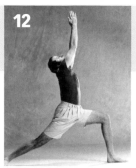

Plank *(p 62)*
3 full breaths

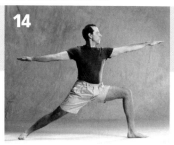

Upward Dog *(p 70)*
3 full breaths

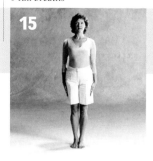

Warrior One *(p 40)*
5 full breaths on each side

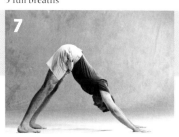

Warrior Two *(p 44)*
5 full breaths on each side

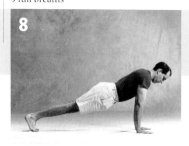

Mountain *(p 36)*
5 full breaths

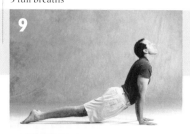

Reverse Triangle *(p 52)*
5 full breaths on each side

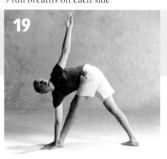

Mountain *(p 36)*
5 full breaths

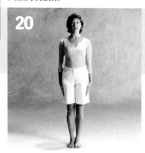

Standing Forward Bend *(p 46)*
5 full breaths

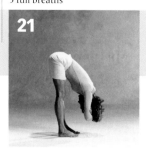

Extended Leg Twist *(p 80)*
5 full breaths on each side

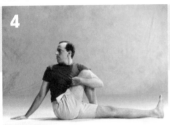

4

Table *(p 62)*
5 full breaths

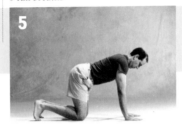

5

Cat *(p 64)*
5 cycles

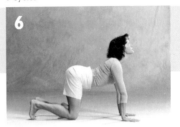

6

Child's Pose *(p 84)*
5 full breaths

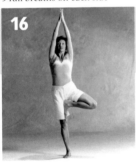

10

Mountain *(p 36)*
5 full breaths

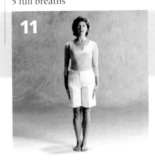

11

Crescent Moon *(p 38)*
5 full breaths on each side

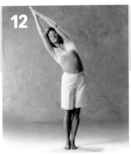

12

Tree *(p 54)*
5 full breaths on each side

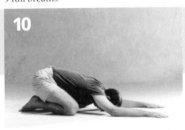

16

Chair *(p 60)*
5 full breaths

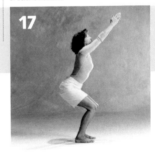

17

Triangle *(p 48)*
5 full breaths on each side

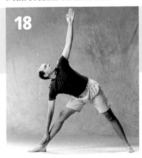

18

Relaxation Pose *(p 94)*
3 minutes plus

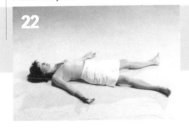

22

Easy Posture *(p 76)*
5 full breaths

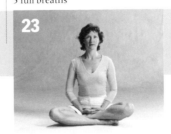

23

DAY 9

Easy Posture (p 76)
5 full breaths

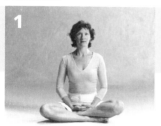

Reclined Knee to Chest (p 92)
5 full breaths on each side

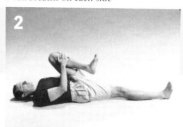

Reclined Ankle to Knee (p 92)
5 full breaths on each side

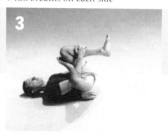

Table (p 62)
5 full breaths

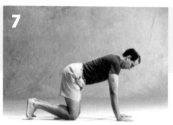

Cat (p 64)
5 cycles

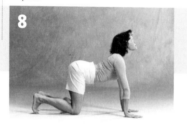

Downward Dog (p 68)
5 full breaths

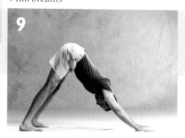

Mountain (p 36)
5 full breaths

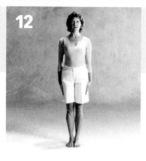

Standing Forward Bend (p 46)
5 full breaths

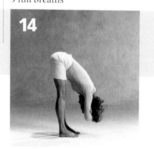

Crescent Moon (p 38)
5 full breaths on each side

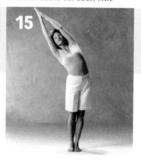

Triangle (p 48)
5 full breaths on each side

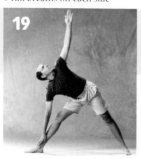

Reverse Triangle (p 52)
5 full breaths on each side

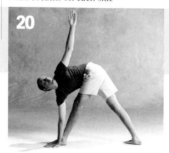

Mountain (p 36)
5 full breaths

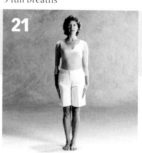

Reclined Twist *(p 92)*
5 full breaths on each side

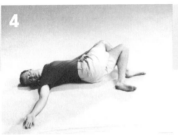

4

Extended Legs Forward Bend *(p 78)*
5 full breaths

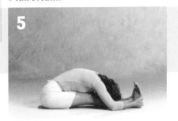

5

Seated Twist *(p 80)*
5 full breaths on each side

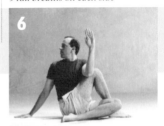

6

Plank *(p 62)*
3 full breaths

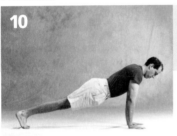

10

Upward Dog *(p 70)*
3 full breaths

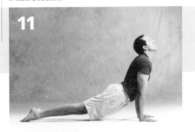

11

Child's Pose *(p 84)*
5 full breaths

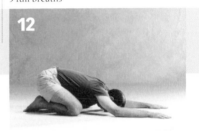

12

Tree *(p 54)*
5 full breaths on each side

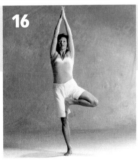

16

Warrior One *(p 40)*
5 full breaths on each side

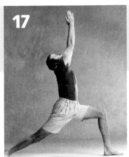

17

Warrior Two *(p 44)*
5 full breaths on each side

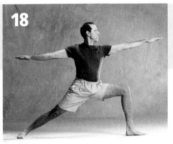

18

Sphinx *(p 86)*
9 full breaths

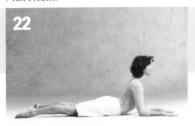

22

Relaxation Pose Knees Up *(p 94)*
3 minutes plus

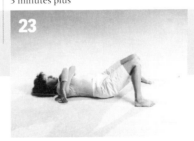

23

Easy Posture *(p 76)*
5 full breaths

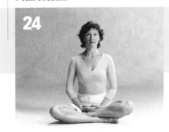

24

DAY 10

Easy Posture (p 76)
5 full breaths

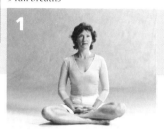

Easy Forward Bend (p 76)
5 full breaths

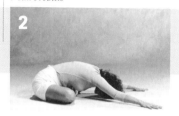

Easy Twist (p 76)
5 full breaths on each side

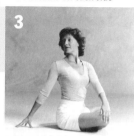

>

Cat (p 64)
5 cycles

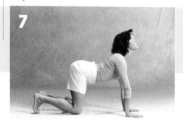

Downward Dog (p 68)
5 full breaths

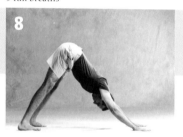

Upward Dog (p 70)
3 full breaths

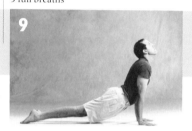

>

Child's Pose (p 84)
5 full breaths

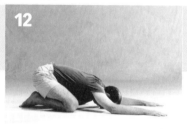

Mountain (p 36)
5 full breaths

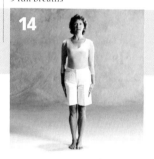

Crescent Moon (p 38)
5 full breaths on each side

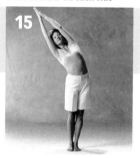

>

Triangle (p 48)
5 full breaths on each side

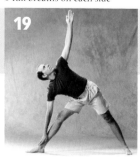

Reverse Triangle (p 52)
5 full breaths on each side

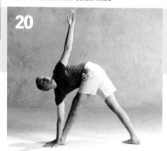

Side Angle (p 56)
5 full breaths on each side

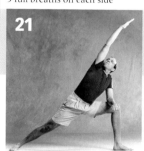

>

Staff *(p 72)*
5 full breaths

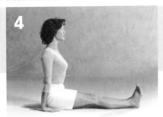

4

Extended Legs Forward Bend *(p 78)*
5 full breaths

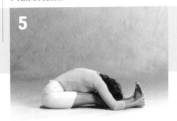

5

Table *(p 62)*
5 full breaths

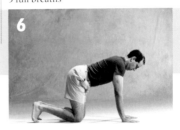

6

Child's Pose *(p 84)*
5 full breaths

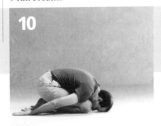

10

Sphinx *(p 86)*
5 full breaths

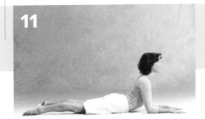

11

Locust *(p 88)*
5 full breaths

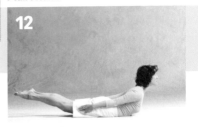

12

Standing Forward Bend *(p 46)*
5 full breaths

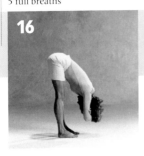

16

Tree *(p 54)*
5 full breaths on each side

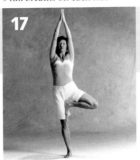

17

Chair *(p 60)*
5 full breaths

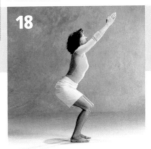

18

Standing Forward Bend *(p 46)*
5 full breaths

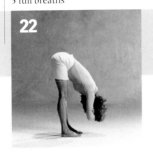

22

Relaxation Pose *(p 94)*
3 minutes plus

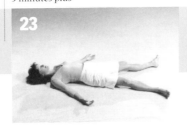

23

Easy Posture *(p 76)*
5 full breaths

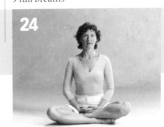

24

DAY 11

Easy Posture (p 76)
5 full breaths

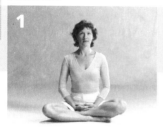

Mountain (p 36)
5 full breaths

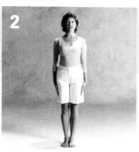

Standing Forward Bend (p 46)
5 full breaths

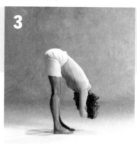

Triangle (p 48)
5 full breaths on each side

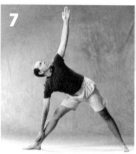

Reverse Triangle (p 52)
5 full breaths on each side

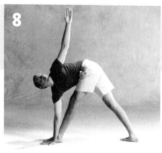

Warrior One (p 40)
5 full breaths on each side

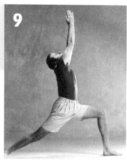

Triangle (p 48)
5 full breaths on each side

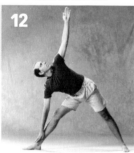

Reverse Triangle (p 52)
5 full breaths on each side

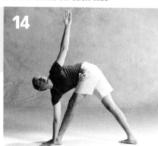

Warrior One (p 40)
5 full breaths on each side

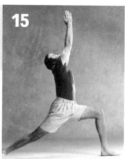

Staff (p 72)
5 full breaths

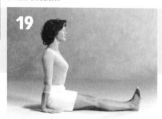

Extended Legs Forward Bend (p 78)
5 full breaths

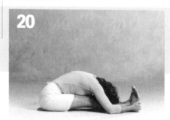

Seated Twist (p 80)
5 full breaths on each side

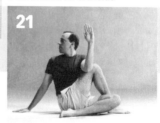

Crescent Moon *(p 38)*
5 full breaths on each side

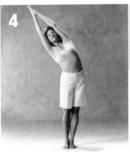

Tree *(p 54)*
5 full breaths on each side

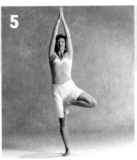

Side Angle *(p 56)*
5 full breaths on each side

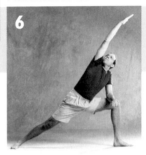

Warrior Two *(p 44)*
5 full breaths on each side

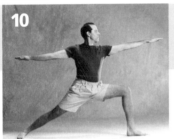

Chair *(p 60)*
5 full breaths

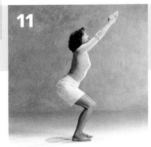

Side Angle *(p 56)*
5 full breaths on each side

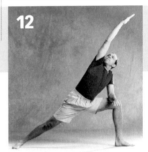

Warrior Two *(p 44)*
5 full breaths on each side

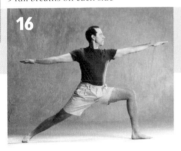

Mountain *(p 36)*
5 full breaths

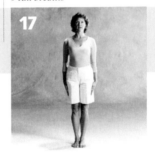

Standing Forward Bend *(p 46)*
5 full breaths

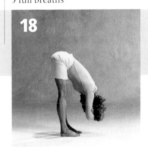

Relaxation Pose *(p 94)*
3 minutes plus

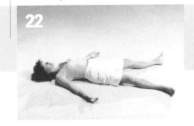

Easy Posture *(p 76)*
5 full breaths

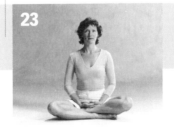

DAY 12

Easy Posture (p 76)
5 full breaths

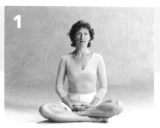
1

Reclined Knee to Chest (p 92)
5 full breaths on each side

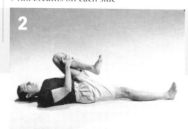
2

Reclined Ankle to Knee (p 92)
5 full breaths on each side

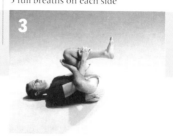
3

Child's Pose (p 84)
5 full breaths

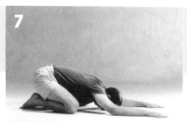
7

Cat (p 64)
5 cycles

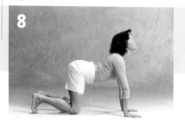
8

Downward Dog (p 68)
5 full breaths

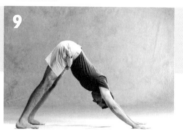
9

Mountain (p 36)
5 full breaths

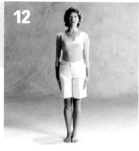
12

Crescent Moon (p 38)
5 full breaths on each side

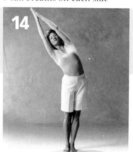
14

Standing Forward Bend (p 46)
5 full breaths

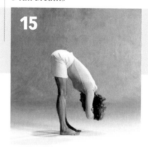
15

Triangle (p 48)
5 full breaths on each side

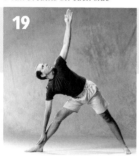
19

Reverse Triangle (p 52)
5 full breaths on each side

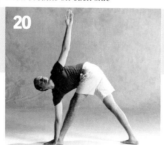
20

Side Angle (p 56)
5 full breaths on each side

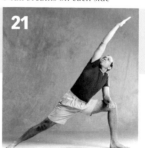
21

>

Reclined Twist *(p 92)*
5 full breaths on each side

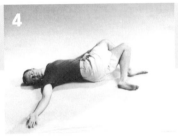

Sphinx *(p 86)*
9 full breaths

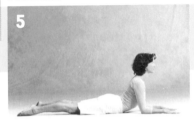

Locust *(p 88)*
5 full breaths

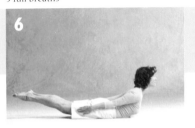

Plank *(p 62)*
3 full breaths

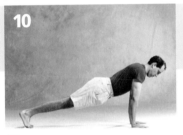

Upward Dog *(p 70)*
3 full breaths

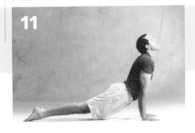

Table *(p 62)*
5 full breaths

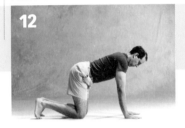

Tree *(p 54)*
5 full breaths on each side

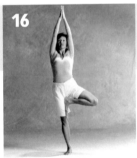

Warrior One *(p 40)*
5 full breaths on each side

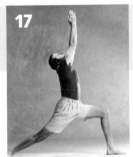

Warrior Two *(p 44)*
5 full breaths on each side

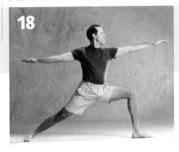

Mountain *(p 36)*
5 full breaths

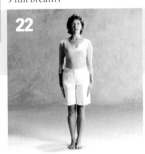

Relaxation Pose *(p 94)*
3 minutes plus

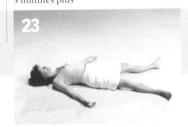

Easy Posture *(p 76)*
5 full breaths

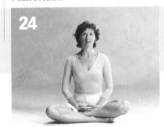

129

DAY 13

Easy Posture (p 76)
5 full breaths

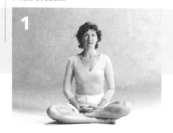

1

Staff (p 72)
5 full breaths

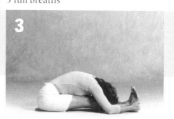

2

Extended Legs Forward Bend (p 78)
5 full breaths

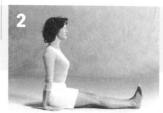

3

Tree (p 54)
5 full breaths on each side

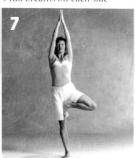

7

Side Angle (p 56)
5 full breaths on each side

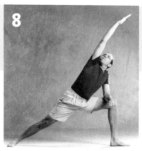

8

Warrior One (p 40)
5 full breaths on each side

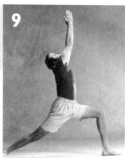

9

Chair (p 60)
5 full breaths

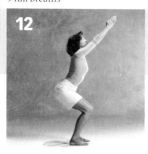

12

Side Angle (p 56)
5 full breaths on each side

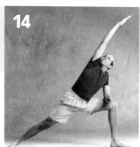

14

Warrior One (p 40)
5 full breaths on each side

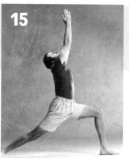

15

Downward Dog (p 68)
5 full breaths

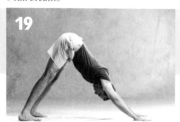

19

Plank (p 62)
3 full breaths

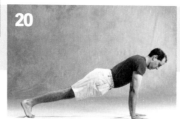

20

Upward Dog (p 70)
3 full breaths

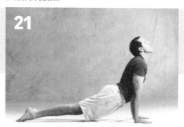

21

Mountain *(p 36)*
5 full breaths

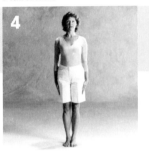

4

Standing Forward Bend *(p 46)*
5 full breaths

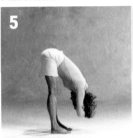

5

Crescent Moon *(p 38)*
5 full breaths on each side

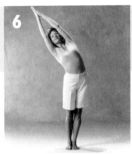

6

Warrior Two *(p 44)*
5 full breaths on each side

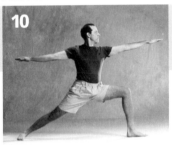

10

Triangle *(p 48)*
5 full breaths on each side

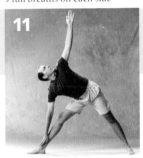

11

Reverse Triangle *(p 52)*
5 full breaths on each side

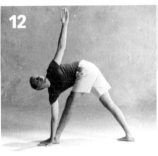

12

Warrior Two *(p 44)*
5 full breaths on each side

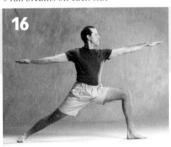

16

Mountain *(p 36)*
5 full breaths

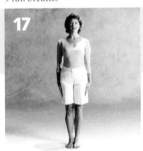

17

Standing Forward Bend *(p 46)*
5 full breaths

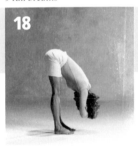

18

Child's Pose *(p 84)*
5 full breaths

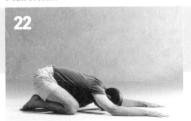

22

Relaxation Pose *(p 94)*
3 minutes plus

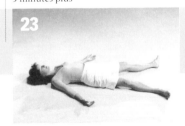

23

Easy Posture *(p 76)*
5 full breaths

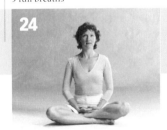

24

DAY 14

Easy Posture (p 76)
5 full breaths

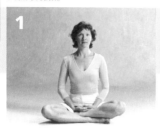

1

Easy Forward Bend (p 76)
5 full breaths

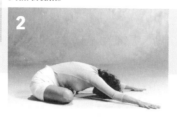

2

Easy Twist (p 76)
5 full breaths on each side

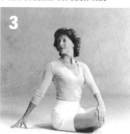

3

Downward Dog (p 68)
5 full breaths

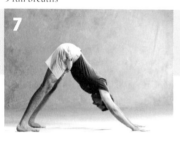

7

Upward Dog (p 70)
3 full breaths

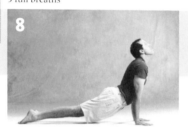

8

Child's pose (p 84)
5 full breaths

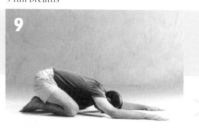

9

Tree (p 54)
5 full breaths on each side

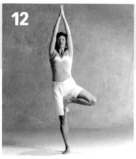

12

Side Angle (p 56)
5 full breaths on each side

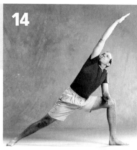

14

Warrior One (p 40)
5 full breaths on each side

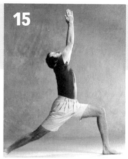

15

Standing Forward Bend (p 46)
5 full breaths

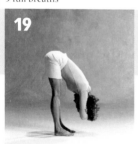

19

Sphinx (p 86)
9 full breaths

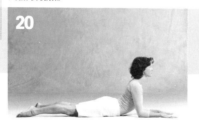

20

Locust (p 88)
5 full breaths

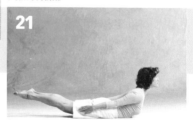

21

Extended Legs Forward Bend (p 78)
5 full breaths

4

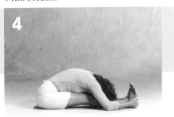

Seated Twist (p 84)
5 full breaths on each side

5

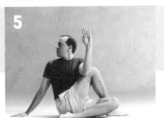

Cat (p 64)
5 cycles

6

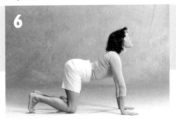

Mountain (p 36)
5 full breaths

10

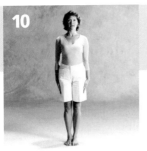

Crescent Moon (p 38)
5 full breaths on each side

11

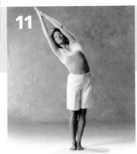

Standing Forward Bend (p 46)
5 full breaths

12

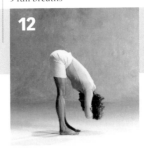

Warrior Two (p 44)
5 full breaths on each side

16

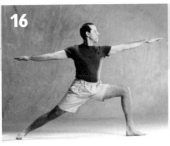

Triangle (p 48)
5 full breaths on each side

17

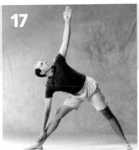

Reverse Triangle (p 52)
5 full breaths on each side

18

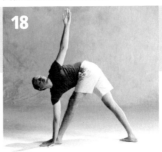

Child's Pose (p 84)
5 full breaths

22

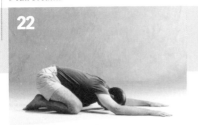

Relaxation Pose (p 94)
3 minutes plus

23

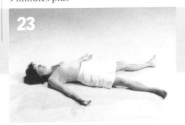

Easy Posture (p 76)
5 full breaths

24

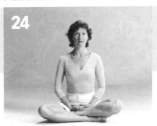

SPECIAL SHORT SESSIONS

Wake-Up

Reclined Knee to Chest *(p 92)*
5 full breaths on each side

Reclined Ankle to Knee *(p 92)*
5 full breaths on each side

Reclined Twist *(p 92)*
5 full breaths on each side

Staff *(p 72)*
5 full breaths

Extended Legs Forward Bend *(p 36)*
5 full breaths

Extended Leg Twist *(p 80)*
5 full breaths on each side

Mountain *(p 36)*
5 full breaths

Standing Forward Bend *(p 46)*
5 full breaths

Crescent Moon *(p 38)*
5 full breaths on each side

Side Angle *(p 56)*
5 full breaths on each side

Mountain *(p 36)*
5 full breaths

Easy Posture *(p 76)*
5 full breaths

Energy

Mountain *(p 36)*
5 full breaths

Crescent Moon *(p 38)*
5 full breaths on each side

Side Angle *(p 56)*
5 full breaths on each side

Warrior One *(p 40)*
5 full breaths on each side

Warrior Two *(p 44)*
5 full breaths on each side

Triangle *(p 48)*
5 full breaths on each side

Reverse Triangle *(p 52)*
5 full breaths on each side

Chair *(p 60)*
5 full breaths

Mountain *(p 36)*
5 full breaths

Standing Forward Bend *(p 46)*
5 full breaths

Downward Dog (p 68)
5 full breaths

Child's Pose *(p 84)*
5 full breaths

Easy Posture *(p 76)*
1 minute or more

Pre-Golf
at the Course

Mountain *(p 36)*
5 full breaths

Standing Forward Bend *(p 46)*
5 full breaths

Crescent Moon *(p 38)*
5 full breaths on each side

Tree Preparation *(p 54)*
5 full breaths on each side

Triangle *(p 48)*
5 full breaths on each side

Reverse Triangle *(p 52)*
5 full breaths on each side

Side Angle *(p 56)*
5 full breaths on each side

Chair *(p 60)*
5 full breaths

Standing Forward Bend *(p 46)*
5 full breaths

Mountain *(p 36)*
5 full breaths

Concentration

Easy Posture *(p 76)*
9 full breaths

Staff *(p 72)*
5 full breaths

Extended Legs Forward Bend *(p 78)*
9 full breaths

Extended Leg Twist *(p 80)*
5 full breaths on each side

Mountain *(p 36)*
5 full breaths

Tree *(p 54)*
5 full breaths one each side

Triangle *(p 48)*
5 full breaths on each side

Reverse Triangle *(p 52)*
5 full breaths on each side

Tree *(p 54)*
5 full breaths on each side

Mountain *(p 36)*
9 full breaths

Easy Posture *(p 76)*
9 full breaths

For the Back

Easy Posture *(p 76)*
5 full breaths

Easy Forward Bend *(p 76)*
5 full breaths

Table *(p 62)*
5 full breaths

Cat *(p 64)*
5 cycles

Child's Pose *(p 84)*
5 full breaths

Mountain *(p 36)*
5 full breaths

Crescent Moon *(p 38)*
5 full breaths on each side

Standing Forward Bend *(p 46)*
5 full breaths

Table *(p 62)*
5 full breaths

Sphinx *(p 86)*
9 full breaths

Locust Alternate Arms *(p 88)*
5 breaths on each side

Child's Pose *(p 84)*
5 full breaths

Easy Twist *(p 76)*
5 full breaths on each side

Relaxation Pose Knees Up *(p 94)*
3 minutes plus

End of the Day Unwind

Easy Posture *(p 76)*
5 full breaths

Easy Forward Bend *(p 76)*
5 full breaths

Easy Twist *(p 76)*
5 full breaths on each side

Staff *(p 72)*
5 full breath

Extended Legs Forward Bend *(p 78)*
5 full breaths

Extended Leg Twist *(p 80)*
5 full breaths on each side

Sphinx *(p 86)*
9 full breaths

Child's Pose *(p 84)*
5 full breaths

Reclined Knee to Chest *(p 92)*
5 full breaths on each side

Reclined Ankle to Knee *(p 92)*
5 full breaths on each side

Reclined Twist *(p 92)*
5 full breaths on each side

Relaxation Pose *(p 94)*
5 minutes plus

Courses beckon,
the land unfolds, challenges,
possibilities await,
surprises, defeats, triumphs.

Thoughts, hopes, plans
set in motion, swings
that make us smile or grimace.
Leaving us loyal and sure, or
groaning, threatening an exit from these
fields of green finally and forever.

The first tee, the maternity ward of our game
where new births are just a swing away.
Is the breath easy? Or do you need
a slap on the back to really let go?
But hopefully not to scream like the newborn,
"Fore!"

The game plays with us as we play it.
We sink a putt and our spirits rise.
We swing easier and the ball travels farther.
Release out to the right and the ball moves left.
The mind boggles, but still
we return.

In wind that moves the ball
or calm like a neutral canvas,
in chill that makes us hesitate
or in warmth that invites thirty-six,
early before all the pins are placed,
or late as the Sun ends the round
the course calls us.

To tests, to tease, to explore one more time.
To walk alone or with friends,
under the sky, into the fields, out into that journey,
that always brings us back to start again.

D.G.

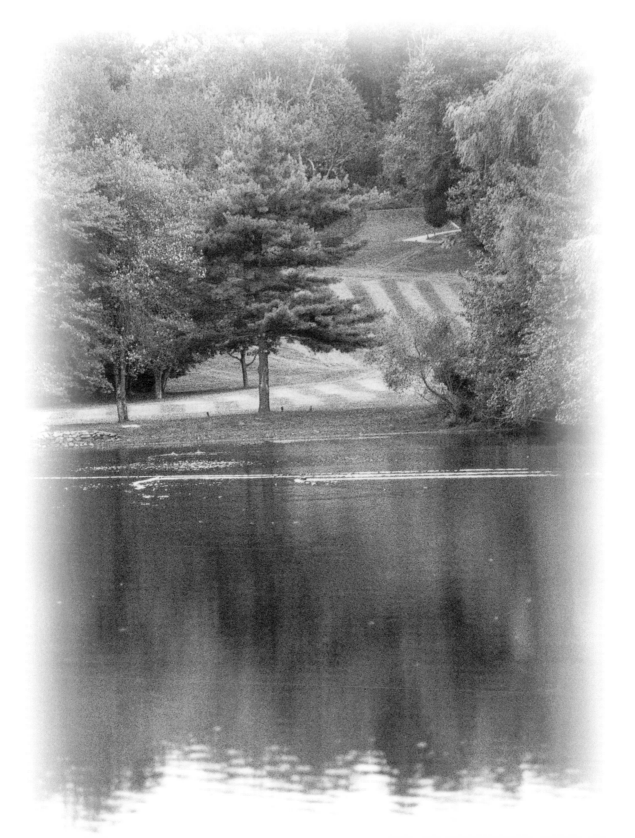

Index

Photography Credits

All studio photographs,
Jim Galante.

Talking Stick Golf Club, Scottsdale,
AZ, North course Hole #16, Dick
Durrance Photography, pg. 42-43.

Waikoloa Beach Resort, King's
Course Hole #2, Kohala Coast,
Hawaii, Dick Durrance
Photography, pg. 49-50.

The Ridge at Castle Pines North,
Hole #18, Castle Rock, CO,
Travis/Tuggle Photography,
pg. 58-59.

Fish Creek Golf Club, Hole #11,
Houston, TX, Dick Durrance
Photography, pg. 66-67.

Whirlwind Golf Club, Hole #7,
Phoenix (Gila River), AZ, pg. 82-83.

Monarch Beach Golf Links,
Hole #3, Dana Point, CA, Graphic
Links Photography, pg. 90-91.

Troon North Golf Club, Pinnacle
Course, Hole #7, Scottsdale, AZ,
Graphic Links Photography,
pg. 98-99.

Rockrimmon Country Club,
Holes #6 and 9, Stamford, CT,
pg. 74-75, 136; back cover and
photographs of the golf swing,
Brad Benjamin.

Acknowledgements

Thanks to my friends with whom I have shared yoga and golf. Thanks to the people I have instructed whom I have learned so much from in the process. Thanks to everybody at Rockrimmon for the friendships and competition. Thanks to Dad for his example of perseverance. Thanks to my late Mom, who among other things, brought a yoga book into the house when I was about four years old. Thanks to Shelley Lynne Cummins, for being the model and for being a friend. Thanks to Jim Galante for the excellent studio photographs. Thanks to Don and Amba Stapelton who understand how you approach teaching is as important as what you teach. Thanks to Troon Golf for sharing some beautiful golf course photographs from their gallery of courses. Thanks to Brad Benjamin for riding around on a cool day and getting a few cool shots too. Thanks to Martin Davis for his inspired suggestion for the cover. Many thanks to Carol Petro for her design work. Thanks to the yoga teacher I met in 1985 who shed so much light on the way. Lastly, and certainly not least, thanks to the reader who has chosen to explore.